THE
LIVING HEART
GUIDE TO
EATING OUT

MICHAEL E. DeBAKEY, M.D.
ANTONIO M. GOTTO, JR., M.D., D.PHIL.
LYNNE W. SCOTT, M.A., R.D./L.D.
With
Mary C. McMann, M.P.H., R.D./L.D.
Suzanne Jaax, M.A., R.D./L.D.
and Danièle Brauchi, R.D./L.D.
Edited by Mary C. McMann

THE
LIVING HEART
GUIDE TO
EATING OUT

A MasterMedia Book
New York

Published by MasterMedia Limited.

MASTERMEDIA and colophon are registered trademarks of MasterMedia Limited.

Designed by Jacqueline Schuman
Production services by Martin Cook Associates, Ltd., New York
Manufactured in the United States of America
10 9 8 7 6 5 4 3 2 1

CONTENTS

---

4   FAST FOOD   *94*

---

5   AIRLINE AND CRUISE SHIP CUISINE   *138*

ACKNOWLEDGMENTS

It was a pleasure to work with so many people who enjoy eating out and are knowledgeable about the preparation of food in restaurants. We are very grateful to Angi Stewart for managing the letters and contacts to fast food companies and airlines and for her patience and excellence in typing the manuscript. We especially appreciate Myrthala Miranda-Guzman for analyzing recipes for the American and several of the ethnic cuisines and for her special contributions to the Mexican food section. We thank Myrthala and Kay Zercher for entering the fast food data into the computer.

We especially want to thank our many friends who shared with us their expertise in ethnic cuisines: Molly Gee (Chinese); Olivier Ciesielski at La Colombe D'Or in Houston (French); Judy Brotherton, John Katsiamakas at Omonia, and Vassili Maqazis at The Great Greek in Houston (Greek); Ajoy Bhattacharya at Bombay Palace in Houston and Suneeta Vaswani (Indian); Paul Hill and Ed Moise at Nino's and Eugene Hinesley, Jr., at the Olive Garden in Houston (Italian); George Hirasaki (Japanese); and Marty Chuenpreecha at Patu and Benzi Vachira at Mai Thai in Houston (Thai).

We very much appreciate the help of David St. John-Grubb, Catharine Powers, and Mary Donovan at the Culinary Institute of America for their valuable suggestions. We are also very grateful to Cathleen Huck, director and archivist at the Conrad N. Hilton Archive and Library, for her help in locating resource material for this book.

We are very grateful to our consultants—Linda McDonald from Houston, Ruth Johnson from California, and Patricia Snyder from Minnesota. We also thank Scott Cornman for his editorial suggestions.

A special thank you goes to Susan Stautberg, president of MasterMedia, for her interest in a book on eating out and for creatively promoting the two editions of our previous book with her. Working with Susan, our enthusiastic and innovative publisher, continues to be an invigorating and rewarding experience.

We wish to thank the many restaurants that shared their menus with us and the fast food companies and airlines that sent information to us.

The Living Heart series of books now spans more than 15 years. First was *The Living Heart* (1977), which answered many of the questions about heart disease asked by patients and their families. New knowledge about treatment of heart disease in the 1970s and early 1980s emphasized the importance of diet. In 1984 we published *The Living Heart Diet,* which appeared on the *New York Times* best-seller list and continues to be a popular book for people interested in changing their eating habits to promote a living heart.

In the 1980s, public interest in heart-healthy food fueled an unprecedented growth in the development of low-fat foods. In 1992 we published *The Living Heart Brand Name Shopper's Guide,* which contained information on calories, fat, saturated fat, cholesterol, and sodium for more than 5,000 foods. The popularity of this book (more than 441,000 copies printed in one year) led to a revised and updated version in 1993. *The Living Heart Brand Name Shopper's Guide,* Revised and Updated, has information on more than 6,100 foods; new regulations for food labeling; identification of foods appropriate for diabetics; chapters on weight control, diabetes, and hypertension; and an update on diet and heart disease.

The growing number of people eating out has increased public interest in selecting lower-fat restaurant foods. In response to this need, we have developed *The Living Heart Guide to Eating Out* to provide practical information to help you select heart-healthy food and increase your eating enjoyment away from home.

The Authors

The Living Heart Guide to Eating Out is a complete guide to heart-healthy eating away from home. This book meets the needs of health-conscious diners by providing suggestions for the wise selection of food in all types of restaurants—from fast food to fine dining—both for travelers and for people dining locally in American restaurants and in ethnic restaurants. *The Living Heart Guide to Eating Out* was written in response to two national trends:

1. More people are eating out more often.
2. An increasing number of people are adopting a heart-healthy eating style.

Surveys show that a typical American (eight years of age and older) eats away from home 3.8 meals per week, or about 198 meals per year. In the United States, 51% of the adults eat at a fast food restaurant and 42% eat at a moderate-priced family restaurant at least once a week. Eating out is big business: in 1970 sales of food in restaurants and other eating places totaled $21.6 billion, and it is estimated that these sales will reach $173.6 billion—an eightfold increase—in 1993.

Americans eat away from home for a number of reasons. Eating out provides an opportunity to choose from a wider variety of foods, an occasion for sharing social times with friends and family, and a setting for conducting business. In addition to its convenience—the perfect answer to a lack of time for food preparation at home—eating out can provide pure enjoyment. It is estimated that almost half of the American food dollar is spent on food consumed away from home.

The Living Heart Guide to Eating Out is de-

signed to meet the needs of today's health-conscious diner. It provides practical information on
selecting heart-healthy food in all types of eating
establishments.

Chapter 1

General Guidelines
for Eating Out

The suggestions for selecting foods lower in fat,
saturated fat, cholesterol, and sodium provided in
this book apply to all types of American and ethnic
cuisines, whether eaten in fine restaurants, cafete-
rias, buffets, delicatessens, or fast food places or
on airplanes and ships. These dietary recommendations are designed to help you achieve a total
day's intake with:

- no more than 30% of calories from fat
- less than 10% of calories from saturated fat
- up to 10% of calories from polyunsaturated fat
- 10% to 15% of calories from monounsatura-
  ted fat
- less than 300 milligrams of cholesterol
- sodium in moderation

The "percent of calories" in these dietary recommendations refers to a total day's calories, not
to calories provided by one food or one meal. The
limit on saturated fat is the most important dietary
recommendation to help lower blood cholesterol,
thereby reducing your risk of heart disease. The
most efficient way to reduce saturated fat is to limit
all fat; reducing fat usually also reduces calories.

Since the recommendations for fat and saturated fat are based on a percent of calories, it is
important to know approximately how many calories you need. Pages 146 to 149 in the Appendix
will help you estimate an appropriate calorie level
for your height, frame size, and activity level. Use
this calorie level with the table on page 151 in the
Appendix to determine the maximum grams of fat

and saturated fat allowable each day to achieve the dietary recommendations shown above.

The maximum grams of fat each day can be divided among the meals and snacks that you eat. For example, at an intake of 2,000 calories, 30% of calories from fat is 67 grams per day. Dividing 67 grams of fat evenly among 3 meals allows about 22 grams of fat per meal. However, most people do not eat as much fat at breakfast as they do at the other meals. Eating a breakfast that is almost fat free is a good way to have more fat at lunch and dinner. The following table shows several ways to divide grams of fat among meals and snacks at three calorie levels:

	Breakfast Grams of Fat	**Lunch** Grams of Fat	**Dinner** Grams of Fat	**Snack** Grams of Fat
Breakfast with negligible fat; all fat divided between lunch and dinner:				
1,500-calorie	0	25	25	0
2,000-calorie	0	33	33	0
2,500-calorie	0	41	41	0
5% of fat at breakfast, 40% at lunch, 50% at dinner, and 5% at evening snack:				
1,500-calorie	3	20	24	3
2,000-calorie	3	27	34	3
2,500-calorie	4	33	42	4
10% of fat at breakfast, 40% at lunch, 45% at dinner, and 5% at evening snack:				
1,500-calorie	5	20	23	2
2,000-calorie	7	27	30	3
2,500-calorie	8	33	38	4
20% of fat at breakfast, 40% at lunch, and 40% at dinner:				
1,500-calorie	10	20	20	0
2,000-calorie	13	27	27	0
2,500-calorie	17	33	33	0

The table shows the maximum grams of fat per day at each calorie level; if you wish to estimate the maximum grams of saturated fat, divide the grams of fat by 3.

The following chapters contain tables providing estimates of calories and values for fat, saturated fat, and cholesterol for foods commonly served in different types of eating places. The tables include both high-fat and low-fat menu items for American foods (beginning on page 10), ethnic foods (see pages 50, 54, 59, 64, 68, 73, 78, 82, 87, 92), and fast foods (beginning on page 96). By using the table above to estimate how much fat to allow yourself per meal, you can plan your fat intake more carefully. For example, at a 2,000-calorie intake, with half the total fat (or 33 grams) allowed for the dinner meal, if you choose veal parmigiana (containing 32 grams of fat), you would need to select a salad with fat-free dressing and plain Italian bread instead of garlic bread. If, however, fettuccine Alfredo (40 grams of fat) is your favorite Italian meal, you need to select other foods at both lunch and dinner that are low in fat in order to compensate for the fat in the fettuccine Alfredo. A second approach could be to split an order of fettuccine Alfredo with your dining companion; the half serving provides about 20 grams of fat, allowing you to add a salad with low-calorie Italian dressing and a bowl of minestrone soup. Another, even better, suggestion is to order an entrée that is lower in fat, such as linguine with red clam sauce (12 grams of fat).

BEFORE YOU EAT OUT

There are a number of things to consider in making dining out an enjoyable heart-healthy experience. The first is what you say to yourself about eating out. You may find yourself choosing high-fat foods and using the excuse that "this is a special occasion" or "it can't hurt to eat deep-fried foods once in a while." Or you may say "I don't eat out that often." If you eat lunch out five days out of seven and dine out in the evening several times each week, eating out is a major contributor to your food intake. Another common thought is that "cleaning your plate is getting your money's worth"; however, it is poor economics to eat more than you want or need.

Americans enjoy an almost unlimited choice of places to eat out. The type of eating establishment you choose will depend on a number of factors: the type of food you prefer, the size of meal you want, the location of a particular restaurant, the amount of time available for the meal, the type of service you favor (fine dining, salad bar, takeout, etc.), and the amount of money you wish to spend.

- Plan ahead. Choose lower-fat foods for other meals and snacks when you are going to eat out to compensate for higher fat levels in restaurant foods.
- Don't skip meals in anticipation of eating out; you will be hungrier and more likely to overeat.
- Choose a place to eat that offers a wide variety of foods. Table-service restaurants with a varied menu give more choices than specialty establishments with limited menus, such as steakhouses, barbecue restaurants, and pizza parlors.

FINDING FAT AND SODIUM IN RESTAURANT FOODS

Fat in food can either be visible or invisible. Invisible fat is found in fatty meats (prime rib, hamburger meat, sausage, and luncheon meats), poultry skin, whole milk, cream, cheese, and desserts (pie, cake, cookies, and ice cream). Sources of visible fat include margarine, butter, oil, mayonnaise, salad dressings, and all fried foods. Although some eating establishments are reducing the fat used in food preparation, most restaurant foods not only are prepared with fat but often are served with high-fat accompaniments, such as cheese, sour cream, melted butter, or rich sauces.

The following menu terms can help you identify foods that are prepared with very little or no added fat.

```
┌─────────────────────────────────────────┐
│        MENU TERMS INDICATING             │
│        LITTLE OR NO FAT USED             │
│         IN FOOD PREPARATION              │
│   • baked                                │
│   • broiled dry (without added fat)      │
│   • grilled                              │
│   • poached                              │
│   • roasted                              │
│   • steamed                              │
│   • tomato sauce                         │
└─────────────────────────────────────────┘
```

The following food names and descriptive terms, commonly used on menus, indicate that a food is high in fat and saturated fat.

```
┌─────────────────────────────────────────┐
│      MENU TERMS INDICATING A FOOD        │
│     HIGH IN FAT AND SATURATED FAT        │
│   • au gratin                            │
│   • basted                               │
│   • braised                              │
│   • buttered/butter sauce/buttery        │
│   • casserole                            │
│   • cheese sauce                         │
│   • creamed/cream sauce/creamy           │
│   • crispy                               │
│   • escalloped/scalloped                 │
│   • fried/deep-fried                     │
│   • gravy/in its own gravy               │
│   • hash                                 │
│   • hollandaise                          │
│   • pan-fried                            │
│   • Parmesan                             │
│   • potpie                               │
│   • prime (the grade of meat with the most fat) │
│   • sautéed                              │
│   • stewed                               │
│   • stuffed                              │
└─────────────────────────────────────────┘
```

Restaurant foods that are low in fat are not necessarily low in sodium: for example, lean ham and dill pickles are both high in sodium. Foods can be high in sodium due either to the sodium present in ingredients, such as cheese, sausage, and soy sauce, or to the salt added in food preparation. The food tables in this book do not include values for sodium, because an accurate estimate of sodium is impossible. Some recipes say "salt to taste," and many ethnic recipes call for ingredients or commercial sauces for which the sodium content is not available.

MENU TERMS INDICATING A FOOD HIGH IN SODIUM

- **broth or au jus (although these terms can mean served with juices from cooking, many restaurants use a prepared meat base that is high in sodium)**
- **cocktail sauce**
- **pickled**
- **smoked**
- **soy sauce and teriyaki sauce**
- **tomato base**

SPECIAL REQUESTS

Most chefs want to please their customers and are usually willing to make requested changes in menu items to ensure that customers enjoy their meal. In a recent survey, almost 70% of restaurant owners said that it is no problem for a customer to ask for a change in a menu item. A survey by the National Restaurant Association showed that more than nine out of ten restaurants would gladly agree to serve sauce and salad dressing on the side; to prepare foods with vegetable oil or margarine instead of butter, lard, or shortening; to broil or bake an entrée rather than fry it; to remove the skin on chicken before cooking it; and to cook without salt when requested. Some foods cannot be changed upon request because they are prepared ahead of time. Examples include soups, sauces, casseroles, cornbread, crêpe fillings, and baked desserts. Fortunately, many foods can be changed, primarily those that are cooked at the time they are ordered.

However, many customers are reluctant to request menu substitutions or to make special requests about food preparation. Calling ahead to the restaurant gives these customers an excellent opportunity to ask the chef or maître d' which foods are low in fat, whether the restaurant can accommodate special requests, and what ingredients are present in specific foods. (The best time to call most restaurants is between 3:30 and 5:30 P.M.) Here are some sample questions you can ask about restaurant food, either when calling ahead or when ordering:

- Which menu items can be modified to reduce fat and/or sodium?
- Is the fat trimmed off before meat is cooked?
- Is the skin removed before chicken is cooked?
- What type of fat (if any) is used in cooking a specific entrée?
- Does a particular entrée include sauce or gravy?
- Are the cooked vegetables seasoned with butter?
- Which sauces have the least amount of fat?
- Is butter or margarine served at the table? If butter, can margarine be requested?

You may find it useful to obtain a copy of the menu before you visit a restaurant. Many restaurants now have fax machines and can provide a copy of their menu immediately. Access to the menu allows you to study the dishes being offered and consider the options available.

> **It is important to remember that, as the paying customer, you should not be afraid to ask for exactly what you want, and you should expect to get it—you deserve the best!**

Chapter 2

American Cuisine

Many foods typically seen in American restaurants have been adapted from favorite ethnic cuisines; examples include pizza, enchiladas, lasagna, croissants, and French bread. These foods, combined with dishes that originated in the United States, make up American cuisine. This chapter includes general guidelines for choosing lower-fat foods in all types of American restaurants; it provides estimates of the calories, fat, saturated fat, and cholesterol in popular American foods eaten at breakfast and brunch and for lunch and dinner. The section on snacks is on page 44, and fast food (which is very American) begins on page 94.

BREAKFAST AND BRUNCH

Food eaten at breakfast can be an important contribution to your day's food intake. If you eat lunch or dinner away from home on a regular basis, consider compensating for the fat in restaurant food by making breakfast an almost fat-free meal; it is easy to do, even when you are eating out. If brunch replaces your breakfast and lunch, the grams of fat allocated to these two meals can be combined (see page 2).

**TIPS ON ORDERING
LOWER-FAT FOOD
AT BREAKFAST OR BRUNCH**

• **Ask for low-fat or skim milk as a beverage, for cereal, and in coffee (instead of cream).**

Tips on Ordering Lower-Fat Food at Breakfast or Brunch (*continued*)

- Request that butter or margarine not be added to grits or cooked cereals.
- Select dry cereal rather than granola, which is usually high in fat.
- Order toast, English muffins, or bagels "dry," with margarine served on the side. Then use a small amount of margarine at the table (it will probably be less than would be added in the kitchen). Waiting until the bread cools slightly before adding margarine decreases the amount that is absorbed. Or skip the margarine and use jam or jelly instead.
- Order pancakes and waffles with fruit topping, syrup, or yogurt topping. If you use margarine, have it served on the side so that you can control the amount used.
- Order a plain poached, a soft-cooked, or a hard-cooked egg (within the recommended limit of 3 egg yolks per week).
- Request that egg substitute or egg whites be used for omelets and scrambled eggs; regular omelets often contain two to three whole eggs. Ask the chef to prepare an egg white and mushroom omelet or a Spanish omelet without cheese and serve it with salsa.
- Select toast and lean ham instead of breakfast sandwiches, which are usually high in calories, fat, saturated fat, and cholesterol because they contain a biscuit or croissant, sausage or bacon, cheese, refried beans, and/or eggs. (See Fast Food, starting on page 94.)
- If you have meat, select lean ham, Canadian bacon, or a breakfast steak instead of bacon or sausage, and count it as part of your meat intake for the day.

```
        TIPS ON LOWERING SODIUM
```
- Select fruit or fruit juice instead of tomato or vegetable juice, which are high in
  sodium.
- Skip meat at breakfast, because even
  lower-fat choices, such as Canadian bacon
  and lean ham, are high in sodium.
- When ordering an omelet (as part of your
  egg allowance), ask that salt and cheese be
  omitted.

The following table gives you an idea of the
calories, fat, saturated fat, and cholesterol content
of selected breakfast and brunch foods. These figures are only estimates, and the content of an
actual dish may vary, depending on how the chef
prepares it. Within each section—fruit and juice,
egg dishes, breads, pancakes and waffles, cereals,
side dishes, and condiments—foods are arranged
from low to high fat. Usually foods lower in fat are
also lower in calories and saturated fat. When the
fat is the same for several foods, those lowest in
calories are listed first.

	Cal	Fat g	Sat g	Chol mg
FRUIT AND JUICE				
Strawberry slices (½ c)	25	0	0	0
Grapefruit (½)	47	0	0	0
Banana (½)	52	0	0	0
Grapefruit juice (1 c)	94	0	0	0
Orange juice (1 c)	112	0	0	0
Apple juice (1 c)	117	0	0	0
Cantaloupe (½)	161	0	0	0
EGG DISHES AND CRÊPES				
Poached egg, no fat added (1)	74	5	2	213
Soft-boiled egg, no fat added (1)	74	5	2	213
Scrambled eggs w/butter (2)	210	17	7	443

	Cal	Fat g	Sat g	Chol mg
Quiche (1/6 of 9")				
w/spinach	333	24	12	139
w/mushroom	347	25	11	158
w/seafood	348	25	12	169
w/bacon	388	29	14	148
Chicken crêpe w/cream sauce (2)	484	25	6	185
Omelet (3 eggs)	353	28	8	675
Florentine (w/spinach)	357	28	13	674
Cheese	432	35	17	695
Ham & cheese	460	36	17	706
Eggs Benedict	404	28	12	278

BAKED GOODS

	Cal	Fat g	Sat g	Chol mg
White or whole-wheat toast, dry (1 sl)	67	1	0	0
Raisin toast, dry (1 sl)	71	1	0	0
English muffin, toasted, dry (1)	133	1	0	0
Bagel, plain (3½" diam)	195	1	0	0
French toast (1 sl)	151	7	2	76
Banana bread (1 sl)	203	7	2	26
Muffin (3" diam)				
Oat	195	8	3	31
Apple or Blueberry	273	12	5	30
Chocolate chip	270	14	6	30
Raisin nut	347	19	6	30
Cinnamon roll (3" diam)	227	9	2	22
Coffeecake, cinnamon w/crunch topping (3" × 3" × 1")	266	9	3	28
Doughnut (1 med)				
Plain cake w/sugar	192	10	2	14
Yeast, glazed	242	14	3	4
w/jelly filling	289	16	4	22
w/creme filling	307	21	6	20
Croissant (1 med)	232	12	7	50
Buttermilk biscuit (3" diam × 1½")	268	12	4	3

c = cup; Cal = calories; Chol = cholesterol; diam = diameter; fl oz = fluid ounce; g = gram; lg = large; mayo = mayonnaise; med = medium; mg = milligram; na = not available; oz = ounce; prep = prepared; Sat = saturated fat; sl = slice; sm = small; Tbsp = tablespoon; tr = trace; tsp = teaspoon; w/ = with; w/o = without

	Cal	Fat g	Sat g	Chol mg
Baked Goods *(continued)*				
Danish pastry (4¼" diam)				
w/fruit	264	13	3	25
w/cheese	266	16	5	30

(See also Breads and Rolls, page 30, and Breads, page 37)

PANCAKES AND WAFFLES

	Cal	Fat g	Sat g	Chol mg
Pancake (4" diam)				
Blueberry (1)	48	2	0	9
Plain (1)	55	2	1	11
Pecan (1)	72	4	1	10
Waffle (9" square)	218	11	2	52

CEREALS

	Cal	Fat g	Sat g	Chol mg
Dry cereal, most types (1 box or about 1 c)	110	1	0	0
Cooked cereal, most brands (1 c)	145	2	0	0
Granola (½ c)	244	11	8	0

SIDE DISHES

	Cal	Fat g	Sat g	Chol mg
Grits, plain (1 c)	141	0	0	0
Canadian bacon (1 sl)	39	2	1	12
Bacon (2 sl)	73	6	2	11
Sausage links (2)	96	8	3	22
Ham slice (3 oz)	192	13	4	53
Sausage patties (2)	199	17	6	43
Hash-brown potatoes (1 c)	297	19	5	0

CONDIMENTS

	Cal	Fat g	Sat g	Chol mg
Jelly (1 Tbsp)	45	0	0	0
Syrup, maple & fruit flavors (1 Tbsp)	55	0	0	0
Honey (1 Tbsp)	64	0	0	0
Margarine (1 pat = 1 tsp)	34	4	1	0
Butter (1 pat = 1 tsp)	34	4	2	10

	Cal	Fat g	Sat g	Chol mg

BEVERAGES

See Beverages, page 41

c = cup; Cal = calories; Chol = cholesterol; diam = diameter; fl oz = fluid ounce; g = gram; lg = large; mayo = mayonnaise; med = medium; mg = milligram; na = not available; oz = ounce; prep = prepared; Sat = saturated fat; sl = slice; sm = small; Tbsp = tablespoon; tr = trace; tsp = teaspoon; w/ = with; w/o = without

Choosing a restaurant in which many of the dishes are cooked to order instead of being prepared ahead of time gives you more control over how food is prepared. The following tips on lower-fat eating in a table-service (sit-down) restaurant apply to many types of eating establishments, ranging from fine dining to neighborhood cafes.

TIPS ON SELECTING
LOWER-FAT FOOD
AT LUNCH AND DINNER

- Read the menu carefully and ask how the food is prepared, paying special attention to terms indicating high fat (see page 5) or high sodium (see page 6).
- Be assertive! Tell your serving person how you want your food prepared.
- To get only the food you want, order "à la carte" instead of ordering a set meal with its accompaniments.
- Don't hesitate to ask for substitutions, such as a baked potato, vegetables, carrot sticks, or a tossed salad instead of French fries; many restaurants do not charge for substitutions if the requested item is on the menu.
- Order two low-fat appetizers in place of an entrée.
- It is considered quite acceptable to request an extra plate and split an entrée at the table with a dinner partner; you may each wish to order a separate salad and vegetables. As a rule, chefs don't like to split an entrée in the kitchen because this labor-intensive task can hold up the production line; also, chefs find it difficult to garnish a "split entrée" and make it look appealing.
- If a restaurant serves large portions, ask for a "to-go bag" so that you can take the uneaten part of your meal home.

> **Tips on Selecting Lower-Fat Food at Lunch and Dinner (*continued*)**
>
> - "Diet plates" are not always low in fat and calories; ask what is included and how the food is prepared.
> - Cafeterias, delicatessens, and buffets allow you to see food before selecting or ordering it. Looking at all the foods being offered before you start down the cafeteria line or place your order in a deli will help you select those that are lower in fat.
> - At a buffet, walk around the table, decide which four or five foods are the lowest in fat, and select those instead of taking some of everything that is offered; do not go back for second helpings.
> - Eat slowly to control the amount of food you consume.
> - Remember, you do not have to clean your plate!

The following table gives you an idea of the calories, fat, saturated fat, and cholesterol content of selected lunch and dinner foods. These figures are only estimates, and the content of an actual dish may vary, depending on how the chef prepares it. Some poultry dishes in the table have values given both with and without skin; some meat dishes have values both with and without fat. Within each section—appetizers and soups, salads and salad bars, entrées, sandwiches, pizza, vegetables, breads, desserts, beverages, and snacks— foods are arranged from low to high fat. Usually foods lower in fat are also lower in calories and saturated fat. When the fat is the same for several foods, those lowest in calories are listed first. If you do not see some of the lower-fat foods listed below on a restaurant menu, you may wish to request them.

	Cal	Fat g	Sat g	Chol mg
APPETIZERS				
Smoked salmon (1 oz)	33	1	0	7
Shrimp cocktail (6 lg shrimp)	70	1	0	80
Prosciutto (½ oz) & honeydew melon (1 sl)	88	2	1	9
Fried zucchini (6 pieces)	105	5	2	34
Mushrooms				
Stuffed and baked (6)	108	8	2	0
Fried (6)	314	16	3	98
Fried calamari (3 oz)	291	14	4	239
Egg rolls (2 med)	215	15	4	57
Fried cheese, 2 pieces (4" × 1" × ¾")	308	18	10	69
Nachos w/beans & cheese (6)	306	20	9	35
Buffalo wings (6)				
Spicy fried chicken wings w/blue cheese dip	328	24	7	90
Fried cauliflower (6)	496	25	4	156
Fried potato skins (2)				
Topped w/cheese, sour cream & bacon	293	26	11	38
Fried eggplant (3 sl)	446	46	12	0

	Cal	Fat g	Sat g	Chol mg
SOUPS				
Chicken noodle (1 c)	82	3	1	5
Minestrone (1 c)	82	3	1	5
Beef w/vegetables (1 c)	83	3	1	5
Green pea (1 c)	164	3	1	0
Tomato bisque (1 c)	160	6	3	17
Black bean (1 c)	168	6	1	2
Lentil (1 c)	169	6	1	2
Bean w/bacon or ham (1 c)	170	6	2	3
Cream of mushroom (1 c)	140	8	4	21
Cream of asparagus (1 c)	143	8	4	21
Cream of broccoli (1 c)	143	8	4	21
Cream of potato (1 c)	153	10	3	7
Manhattan clam chowder (tomato base) (1 c)	220	10	2	34
Cream of chicken (1 c)	192	11	5	27
New England clam chowder (cream base) (1 c)	276	14	5	50
Fish chowder (1 c)	287	14	5	77
Cheese (1 c)	230	15	9	46
Gumbo w/seafood (1 c)	262	16	4	69
Gazpacho (1 c)	191	17	3	0
Oyster stew (1 c)	270	18	6	88
Vichyssoise (chilled potato soup) (1 c)	277	21	13	65

c = cup; Cal = calories; Chol = cholesterol; diam = diameter; fl oz = fluid ounce; g = gram; lg = large; mayo = mayonnaise; med = medium; mg = milligram; na = not available; oz = ounce; prep = prepared; Sat = saturated fat; sl = slice; sm = small; Tbsp = tablespoon; tr = trace; tsp = teaspoon; w/ = with; w/o = without

Many people assume that all foods from a salad bar are low in calories and fat; however, some salad bar selections are high in calories and fat. A salad bar gives you the advantage of selecting specific low-fat foods and controlling the amount of each food.

TIPS ON SELECTING LOWER-FAT SALADS

- Select more fresh vegetables and fruits and fewer prepared salads, such as pasta, chicken, tuna, and potato salad.
- Add a serving of marinated vegetables on top of your salad instead of regular dressing; the marinade will drip throughout and flavor the salad greens.
- Ask if low-calorie salad dressings are available. If you choose regular salad dressing, it can be added to salad in one of three ways: tossed with the salad in the kitchen, added on top of the salad, or served in a side dish. The third option allows you more control of the amount of dressing consumed, unless you tend to eat all that is in the dish; in that case, choose the first option as being potentially lower in fat.

TIPS ON LOWERING SODIUM

- Eat plain raw vegetables instead of pickled vegetables.
- Select fresh vegetables and fruit instead of prepared salads, such as chicken, tuna, potato, and pasta salads, which are higher in sodium.
- Use lemon juice, vinegar, or oil and vinegar (from separate bottles) instead of prepared dressings on salad.

	Cal	Fat g	Sat g	Chol mg
VEGETABLES				
Salad greens (2 c)	29	0	0	0
Cucumber, raw (6 sl)	4	0	0	0
Tomato, cherry (1)	4	0	0	0
Bean sprouts (½ c)	5	0	0	0
Mushrooms, raw (½ c chopped)	9	0	0	0
Broccoli, raw (½ c pieces)	10	0	0	0
Spinach, raw (1 c)	12	0	0	0
Cauliflower, raw (1 c pieces)	24	0	0	0
Beets, sliced (½ c)	26	0	0	0
Carrots, raw (½ c sl)	26	0	0	0
Kidney beans (½ c)	113	0	0	0
Mushroom pieces, marinated (½ c)	29	2	0	0
Green beans, marinated (½ c)	34	2	0	0
Garbanzo beans/chickpeas (½ c)	134	2	0	0
PREPARED SALADS				
Gelatin w/fruit (½ c)	87	0	0	0
Fruit salad, canned (½ c)	93	0	0	0
Pasta salad, no meat or cheese, w/Italian dressing (½ c)	73	3	0	0
Gelatin w/cottage cheese & fruit (½ c)	119	5	3	19
Ambrosia fruit salad (½ c)	127	7	5	15
Pea salad w/cheese & mayo dressing (½ c)	129	8	3	14
Tabouli (½ c)	132	9	1	0
Three-bean salad w/oil dressing (½ c)	143	11	2	0
Carrot & raisin salad w/mayo dressing (½ c)	180	14	2	10

c = cup; Cal = calories; Chol = cholesterol; diam = diameter; fl oz = fluid ounce; g = gram; lg = large; mayo = mayonnaise; med = medium; mg = milligram; na = not available; oz = ounce; prep = prepared; Sat = saturated fat; sl = slice; sm = small; Tbsp = tablespoon; tr = trace; tsp = teaspoon; w/ = with; w/o = without

	Cal	Fat g	Sat g	Chol mg
Prepared Salads *(continued)*				
Chef's salad w/turkey (1 oz), ham (1 oz), Swiss cheese (1 oz) & ½ egg, no dressing	245	14	6	158
Cole slaw w/mayo dressing (½ c)	142	15	2	11
Crab salad w/mayo dressing, no egg (½ c)	170	15	2	41
Shrimp salad w/mayo dressing, no egg (½ c)	179	15	2	79
Potato salad w/mayo dressing (½ c)	212	15	2	11
Macaroni salad w/mayo dressing & egg, no meat or cheese (½ c)	222	15	2	11
Waldorf salad (½ c)	205	19	3	11
Tuna salad w/mayo dressing, no egg (½ c)	279	24	4	24
Chicken salad, w/o egg (½ c)	352	32	5	61

SALAD DRESSINGS

	Cal	Fat g	Sat g	Chol mg
Thousand Island (¼ c)	235	22	4	16
Honey mustard (¼ c)	276	25	4	0
French (¼ c)	268	26	6	36
Italian (¼ c)	275	28	4	0
Low-calorie (¼ c)	63	6	1	4
Vinegar & oil (¼ c)	275	28	4	0
Russian (¼ c)	302	31	4	11
Low-calorie (¼ c)	162	14	2	15
Blue cheese or Roquefort (¼ c)	308	32	6	10

"EVERYTHING ELSE ON THE SALAD BAR"

	Cal	Fat g	Sat g	Chol mg
Pickle, dill (1 lg)	24	0	0	0
Sweet gherkin (1 lg)	41	0	0	0
Bacon bits (1 Tbsp)				
Imitation	32	1	0	0
Real	29	2	1	4
Parmesan cheese (1 Tbsp)	23	2	1	4
Black olive slices (¼ c)	39	4	1	0
Sunflower seeds (1 Tbsp)	46	4	0	0

	Cal	Fat g	Sat g	Chol mg
Croutons (½ c)	88	4	3	0
Cottage cheese, regular or creamed (½ c)	109	5	3	16
Cheddar cheese, grated (¼ c)	114	9	6	30

c = cup; Cal = calories; Chol = cholesterol; diam = diameter; fl oz = fluid ounce; g = gram; lg = large; mayo = mayonnaise; med = medium; mg = milligram; na = not available; oz = ounce; prep = prepared; Sat = saturated fat; sl = slice; sm = small; Tbsp = tablespoon; tr = trace; tsp = teaspoon; w/ = with; w/o = without

Most fish and poultry without skin (cooked without added fat) is lower in fat than red meat. Most fish is naturally low in fat; any fat found in fish is rich in polyunsaturated fat, which does not cause an increase in blood cholesterol levels. Many restaurants greatly increase the amount of fat in meat, poultry, and fish dishes during preparation by sautéing, pan-frying, breading and deep-frying, adding sauce, and basting before and during broiling and grilling. Meat, poultry, and fish that is "broiled" in a restaurant is often cooked with a generous amount of butter or margarine to prevent it from drying out. It is recommended that you eat no more than 6 ounces (oz) (cooked weight) of meat, poultry, and fish per day; 3 oz of meat is the size of a deck of playing cards. Weights of meat, poultry, and fish given on restaurant menus are for the raw meat; allow for 25% weight loss during cooking. (In the following table, weights are given for raw meat.)

TIPS ON ORDERING LOWER-FAT ENTRÉES

- **Select roasted, grilled, or baked meats instead of fried meat or casseroles, which are usually high in fat because of the ground meat, butter, sour cream, oil, and/or cheese in them.**
- **Select lean red meats, such as sirloin or tenderloin of beef, filet mignon (without bacon), loin pork chops, ham steak, or leg of lamb with the fat cut off, rather than higher-fat cuts, such as prime rib, prime steaks, T-bone steaks, rib-eye steaks, or ribs.**
- **Ask that meat fat and poultry skin be removed before cooking.**

Tips on Ordering Lower-Fat Entrées
(*continued*)

- Ask that a very small amount of oil or no oil be used in sautéing or stir-frying foods; request that meat, poultry, and fish be broiled or grilled without added fat.
- Requesting that fish be "broiled dry" may not result in a tasty entrée—instead, ask to have your fish "baked with a splash of wine," "poached," or "shallow poached" (partially cooked on top of stove and finished in the oven).
- Select entrées without rich sauce or cheese, or ask that sauce or gravy for meat, fish, or poultry be served in a side dish so that you can control the amount eaten.

TIPS ON LOWERING SODIUM

- Choose cooked-to-order dishes and ask that they be prepared without salt, MSG (monosodium glutamate), or soy sauce. Sodium in food prepared ahead of time, including soups, sauces, gravies, and casseroles, cannot be reduced.
- Use lemon instead of cocktail or tartar sauce with fish.

	Cal	Fat g	Sat g	Chol mg
FISH AND SHELLFISH				
Broiled flounder, basted w/oil (8 oz)	226	6	2	111
Grilled red snapper, basted w/oil (8 oz)	245	7	2	120
Poached salmon, no fat or sauce (8 oz)	278	11	2	74

c = cup; Cal = calories; Chol = cholesterol; diam = diameter; fl oz = fluid ounce; g = gram; lg = large; mayo = mayonnaise; med = medium; mg = milligram; na = not available; oz = ounce; prep = prepared; Sat = saturated fat; sl = slice; sm = small; Tbsp = tablespoon; tr = trace; tsp = teaspoon; w/ = with; w/o = without

	Cal	Fat g	Sat g	Chol mg
Fish and Shellfish (continued)				
Fried shrimp (6–8)	454	25	5	201
Fried catfish (8 oz)	728	39	7	116

CHICKEN

	Cal	Fat g	Sat g	Chol mg
Grilled chicken breast w/o skin (½ lg breast)	183	6	2	75
w/skin	256	13	4	89
Chicken teriyaki w/o skin (½ lg breast)	198	6	2	75
w/skin	271	13	4	89
Chicken & pasta salad plate	334	21	4	64
Baked chicken half w/o skin	495	22	6	203
w/skin	736	43	12	256
Chicken potpie	439	24	9	46
Fried chicken breast	447	25	7	78
Thigh & drumstick	552	34	9	103

BEEF

	Cal	Fat g	Sat g	Chol mg
Swiss steak (8 oz)	222	9	2	66
Sirloin steak, fat trimmed off (8 oz)	267	10	3	111
Fat eaten	377	24	9	112
Veal steak, fat trimmed off (8 oz)	252	11	4	148
Filet mignon or tenderloin, fat trimmed off (8 oz)	331	17	6	110
Fat eaten	427	27	10	127
London broil w/flank steak, fat trimmed off (8 oz)	373	19	7	124
Fat eaten	458	29	11	136
Beef Stroganoff w/noodles	416	23	10	106
Chili con carne (1½ c)	412	25	10	94
Stuffed green peppers (2)	502	25	10	94
Porterhouse steak, fat trimmed off (16 oz)	541	28	10	180
Fat eaten	804	58	22	206
Swedish meatballs w/sauce (8 oz)	426	29	13	147
Pot roast of beef, fat trimmed off (8 oz)	562	34	13	181
Fat eaten	762	59	24	191

	Cal	Fat g	Sat g	Chol mg
Meat loaf (8 oz)	574	34	13	181
Chopped beefsteak (8 oz)	472	35	14	137
Chicken fried steak (12 oz)	928	53	15	155
w/gravy (¾ c)	1210	75	23	186

PORK

Pork tenderloin (8 oz)	376	11	4	211
Sweet & sour pork (8 oz total)	629	38	11	75

c = cup; Cal = calories; Chol = cholesterol; diam = diameter; fl oz = fluid ounce; g = gram; lg = large; mayo = mayonnaise; med = medium; mg = milligram; na = not available; oz = ounce; prep = prepared; Sat = saturated fat; sl = slice; sm = small; Tbsp = tablespoon; tr = trace; tsp = teaspoon; w/ = with; w/o = without

TIPS ON ORDERING A
LOWER-FAT SANDWICH

- Choose a prepared-to-order sandwich, which allows you more control over ingredients, rather than one prepared ahead of time. Request low-fat toppings, such as lettuce, tomato, pickles, and onion, instead of bacon and cheese (see page 30); bread, a bun, or a roll instead of a croissant (see page 30); and mustard or catsup instead of mayonnaise.
- Select lean roast beef, lean ham, sliced turkey or chicken, or grilled chicken, which are lower in fat than hamburgers or mixed filling sandwiches (tuna, chicken, ham, or egg salad).
- When ordering a hamburger, choose one with a small meat patty and add lettuce, tomato, pickle, and onion instead of selecting one with a large patty or double meat. (Also see Fast Food, page 94.)
- When ordering a submarine or po-boy sandwich, choose turkey, lean ham, or lean roast beef instead of cold cuts, and omit the cheese and the oil-and-vinegar dressing that is usually sprinkled on top.
- Split a large sandwich with a friend by ordering extra bread and sharing the meat.
- Order a deli "lite" sandwich, which usually contains less meat than a regular sandwich.

TIPS ON LOWERING SODIUM

- Select lean roast beef, turkey, or grilled chicken instead of cold cuts and cheese, which are higher in sodium.
- If "fresh" cooked turkey is available, choose it instead of "deli-type" sliced turkey and roast beef, which are processed with sodium.

Sandwich shops and delis vary in the amount of meat or mixed filling (such as pimento cheese, chicken, tuna, egg, and ham salad) they use in a sandwich. A sliced meat sandwich may contain 2 to 7 oz meat, or even more. In the table below, 4 oz sliced meat or 4 oz sandwich filling has been used for cold sandwiches; the amounts of bread and condiments used are the same, to allow easy comparison of the calories, fat, saturated fat, and cholesterol. As you look at the grams of fat in different hot sandwiches, keep in mind that the amount of meat varies. For example, a hot dog is lower in fat than some of the other sandwiches because it contains only 1½ oz meat. The fried fish sandwich gets its fat from the breading, the fat used for frying, and the tartar sauce; it provides only 1½ oz fish. Also note that although an egg salad sandwich is relatively low in fat when compared to many other sandwiches, it provides two to three times the cholesterol. Remember that the meat, poultry, or fish in a sandwich is part of the "no more than 6 oz" meat recommended for the day. In each category, the sandwiches are arranged from low to high fat.

	Cal	Fat g	Sat g	Chol mg
SLICED MEAT OR CHEESE SANDWICHES (4 oz meat, 2 sl bread w/mustard, 1 lettuce leaf & 2 sl tomato)				
Turkey or chicken	272	6	1	48
Ham	352	12	4	69
Roast beef	431	19	7	92
Corned beef	435	24	8	113
Bologna	508	34	13	64
Pastrami	546	35	12	107
Cheese	576	37	23	109
MIXED FILLING SANDWICHES (4 oz filling, 2 sl bread, 1 lettuce leaf & 2 sl tomato)				
Egg salad	353	19	4	331
Ham salad	414	21	5	98
Tuna salad	423	22	4	84
Pimento cheese	395	23	14	69
Chicken salad	455	26	5	117
HOT SANDWICHES				
Steak (3 oz) on a bun	344	11	4	66
Hot dog on a bun (1½ oz weiner)	264	15	5	23
w/chili	334	18	7	35
w/cheese	370	24	11	50
w/chili & cheese	406	26	12	56
Denver or Western w/scrambled egg, chopped ham, onion & green pepper on bread (2 sl)	306	15	4	225
Roast beef (3½ oz) w/gravy on bread (2 sl)	392	16	6	72
Egg (1), cheese (1 oz) & ham (1 oz) on an English muffin	351	17	7	248
Breaded chicken fillet (2 oz) on a bun, plain w/o condiments	388	17	5	48

	Cal	Fat g	Sat g	Chol mg
Bacon (3 sl), lettuce & tomato on bread (2 sl)	323	18	7	30
Breaded fish (1½ oz) w/tartar sauce on a bun	424	19	4	37
Club w/bacon (2 sl), turkey (2 oz), tomato & mayo on bread (3 sl)	483	22	5	65
w/ham (3 oz), cheese (1 oz), tomato & mayo on bread (3 sl)	605	32	12	100
Meatball (3½ oz) & spaghetti sauce on a submarine roll	480	23	8	78
Beef barbecue (3 oz) on a bun	415	24	10	72
Monte Cristo w/ham (1 oz), cheese (1 oz), & bread (2 sl), egg-dipped & fried	423	24	12	172
Grilled cheese (2 oz cheese, 2 sl bread)	413	27	13	55
Gyro w/beef & lamb (5 oz) & condiments in pita bread	546	28	11	126
Reuben w/corned beef (1.3 oz), sauerkraut, cheese (1.3 oz) & dressing on rye bread (2 sl), grilled	543	37	12	79

HAMBURGERS

	Cal	Fat g	Sat g	Chol mg
Hamburger, regular, single meat patty w/catsup, mustard, pickle & onions	275	10	4	43
w/catsup, mustard, mayo, pickle, onions, lettuce & tomato	279	13	4	26
Cheeseburger, regular, single meat patty, plain	320	15	6	50
w/catsup, mustard, mayo, pickles, onions, lettuce & tomatoes	359	20	10	52

c = cup; Cal = calories; Chol = cholesterol; diam = diameter; fl oz = fluid ounce; g = gram; lg = large; mayo = mayonnaise; med = medium; mg = milligram; na = not available; oz = ounce; prep = prepared; Sat = saturated fat; sl = slice; sm = small; Tbsp = tablespoon; tr = trace; tsp = teaspoon; w/ = with; w/o = without

	Cal	Fat g	Sat g	Chol mg
Hamburgers *(continued)*				
Hamburger, double meat patty, plain	544	28	10	99
w/catsup, mustard, pickles & onions	576	32	12	102
Cheeseburger, large, single meat patty, plain	608	33	15	96
w/bacon, catsup, mustard, pickles & onions	609	37	16	112

SPREADS

	Cal	Fat g	Sat g	Chol mg
Mustard (1 Tbsp)	11	0	0	0
Catsup (1 Tbsp)	16	0	0	0
Mayonnaise (1 Tbsp)	99	11	2	8

SANDWICH TOPPINGS

	Cal	Fat g	Sat g	Chol mg
Lettuce leaf (1)	1	0	0	0
Dill pickle spear (1)	5	0	0	0
Onion slice (1)	5	0	0	0
Tomato slices (2)	8	0	0	0
Pickle, sweet (1 med)	18	0	0	0
Mozzarella, part skim (1 sl = 1 oz)	72	5	3	16
Bacon slices (2)	73	6	2	11
Oil & vinegar dressing drizzled over sandwich (1 Tbsp)	69	7	1	0
Provolone cheese (1 sl = 1 oz)	101	8	5	25
Swiss cheese (1 sl = 1 oz)	107	8	5	26
American cheese (1 sl = 1 oz)	106	9	6	27
Cheddar cheese (1 sl = 1 oz)	114	9	6	30

BREADS AND ROLLS

	Cal	Fat g	Sat g	Chol mg
Bread				
White (2 sl)	135	2	0	2
Whole-wheat (2 sl)	139	2	0	2
Pumpernickel & rye (2 sl)	150	2	0	0
Kaiser roll (1 med)	156	2	0	2

| | | Fat | Sat | Chol |
	Cal	g	g	mg
Submarine or hoagie roll (1 med)	290	3	1	3
Croissant (1 lg for sandwich)	406	21	12	88

(See also Baked Goods, page 11,
and Breads, page 37)

c = cup; Cal = calories; Chol = cholesterol; diam = diameter; fl oz
= fluid ounce; g = gram; lg = large; mayo = mayonnaise; med =
medium; mg = milligram; na = not available; oz = ounce; prep =
prepared; Sat = saturated fat; sl = slice; sm = small; Tbsp = tablespoon; tr = trace; tsp = teaspoon; w/ = with; w/o = without

TIPS ON ORDERING LOWER-FAT PIZZA

- Eat a large salad before eating pizza to take the edge off your appetite.
- Order a vegetarian rather than a meat pizza.
- Request that less cheese or no cheese be used.
- If you want meat, request it on half of the pizza. Canadian bacon is usually the leanest type of meat available.
- Order a thin-crust pizza; deep-dish pizza may have extra cheese and meat toppings, making it even higher in fat and saturated fat.

TIPS ON LOWERING SODIUM

- Request that little or no cheese be used on the pizza.
- Select vegetable toppings (except olives), which are lower in sodium than meat toppings.
- Request that anchovies not be added to your pizza.

	Cal	Fat g	Sat g	Chol mg
THIN CRUST (¼ of 14″ pizza)				
Pizza w/o cheese & w/vegetables	265	13	2	2
Cheese pizza	374	20	7	24
w/green pepper	379	20	7	24
w/Canadian bacon	435	23	8	43
w/olives	454	27	8	24
w/1 meat topping (pepperoni, sausage, or hamburger)	535	33	11	60
w/2 meat toppings (pepperoni, sausage, or hamburger)	590	38	13	69
THICK CRUST (¼ of 14″ pizza)				
Pizza w/o cheese & w/vegetables	704	15	2	0
Cheese pizza	879	26	9	34
w/green pepper	883	26	9	34
w/Canadian bacon	939	29	10	53
w/olives	958	34	10	34
w/1 meat topping (pepperoni, sausage, or hamburger)	1040	40	14	70
w/2 meat toppings (pepperoni, sausage, or hamburger)	1094	45	16	79

c = cup; Cal = calories; Chol = cholesterol; diam = diameter; fl oz = fluid ounce; g = gram; lg = large; mayo = mayonnaise; med = medium; mg = milligram; na = not available; oz = ounce; prep = prepared; Sat = saturated fat; sl = slice; sm = small; Tbsp = tablespoon; tr = trace; tsp = teaspoon; w/ = with; w/o = without

---

TIPS ON ORDERING
LOWER-FAT VEGETABLES

- Top a baked potato with chives or green onions, catsup, lemon juice, jalapeño peppers, mustard, salsa, or a small amount of margarine or low-fat ranch or French dressing. Potatoes that are French-fried, creamed, hash-browned, escalloped, au gratin, mashed, stuffed, or twice baked are high in fat.
- Request marinara sauce instead of cream sauce with pasta. Foods with cheese sauce, such as macaroni and cheese, are high in fat.
- Select foods without rich sauce or cheese.

TIPS ON LOWERING SODIUM

- Order vegetables without sauce or cheese.
- Select a baked potato and add green onion, lemon juice, chives, or a small amount of margarine.

	Cal	Fat g	Sat g	Chol mg
BAKED POTATO W/TRIMMINGS				
Baked potato (1 lg)	130	0	0	0
Sour cream (2 Tbsp)	56	6	3	19
Cheese, grated (¼ c)	114	9	2	9
Bacon, crumbled (2 Tbsp)	58	5	2	9
Butter (3 pats)	102	12	7	31
Potato w/all trimmings listed above	460	32	14	68
VEGETABLES SEASONED WITH MARGARINE				
Turnip greens (¾ c)	47	3	1	0
Zucchini (¾ c)	47	3	1	0
Italian style	52	3	1	0
Cabbage (¾ c)	49	3	1	0

	Cal	Fat g	Sat g	Chol mg
Cauliflower (¾ c)	51	3	1	0
Green beans (¾ c)	52	3	1	0
Asparagus (¾ c)	63	3	1	0
Broccoli (¾ c)	64	3	1	0
Spinach (¾ c)	65	3	1	0
Okra, steamed (¾ c)	70	3	1	0
Brussels sprouts (¾ c)	74	3	1	0
Peas & carrots (¾ c)	83	3	1	0
Carrots, glazed (¾ c)	102	3	1	0
Green peas (¾ c)	119	3	1	0
Corn, whole kernel (¾ c)	125	3	1	0
Corn on the cob w/margarine (1 sm)	96	4	1	0
Mashed potatoes (¾ c)	183	6	1	2
Sweet potato, candied (¾ c)	341	8	2	1

VEGETABLES SEASONED WITH BACON OR MEAT

	Cal	Fat g	Sat g	Chol mg
Mustard greens w/bacon (¾ c)	48	3	1	0
Tomatoes & okra w/bacon (¾ c)	66	3	1	2
Black-eyed peas w/bacon (¾ c)	171	3	1	2
Pinto beans w/bacon (¾ c)	198	3	1	2
Baked beans w/pork (¾ c)				
w/franks	274	11	4	26
w/bacon	381	12	4	19

VEGETABLES WITH SAUCE

	Cal	Fat g	Sat g	Chol mg
Spinach, creamed (¾ c)	111	5	1	3
Green peas, creamed (¾ c)	165	5	1	3
Cauliflower w/cheese sauce (¾ c)	123	8	3	15
Asparagus w/cheese sauce (¾ c)	135	8	4	15
Broccoli w/cheese sauce (¾ c)	136	8	3	15
Spinach w/cheese sauce (¾ c)	137	8	3	15
Beets, Harvard (¾ c)	161	9	2	0

c = cup; Cal = calories; Chol = cholesterol; diam = diameter; fl oz = fluid ounce; g = gram; lg = large; mayo = mayonnaise; med = medium; mg = milligram; na = not available; oz = ounce; prep = prepared; Sat = saturated fat; sl = slice; sm = small; Tbsp = tablespoon; tr = trace; tsp = teaspoon; w/ = with; w/o = without

	Cal	Fat g	Sat g	Chol mg
Vegetables with Sauce *(continued)*				
Potatoes au gratin (w/cheese sauce) (¾ c)	245	12	5	21
Green bean casserole w/cheese & cream of mushroom soup (¾ c)	208	13	7	33
Squash casserole w/cheese, milk & margarine (¾ c)	401	29	10	101

FRIED VEGETABLES

	Cal	Fat g	Sat g	Chol mg
Mushrooms sautéed in butter (¾ c)	82	6	4	16
Okra, cornmeal-dipped & fried (¾ c)	125	6	1	38
French fries (¾ c)	128	8	2	0
Mushrooms, batter-dipped & fried (¾ c)	187	9	2	58
Fried onion rings (¾ c)	143	10	2	28

c = cup; Cal = calories; Chol = cholesterol; diam = diameter; fl oz = fluid ounce; g = gram; lg = large; mayo = mayonnaise; med = medium; mg = milligram; na = not available; oz = ounce; prep = prepared; Sat = saturated fat; sl = slice; sm = small; Tbsp = tablespoon; tr = trace; tsp = teaspoon; w/ = with; w/o = without

---

**TIPS ON ORDERING
LOWER-FAT BREADS**

- Select hard rolls, hard breadsticks, saltine crackers, or sliced bread, which are lower in fat than cornbread, muffins, and dinner rolls (brushed with margarine or butter).
- Eat bread, rolls, and crackers without butter or margarine.

TIP FOR LOWERING SODIUM

- Yeast breads, such as sliced bread and hard rolls, are lower in sodium than breads containing baking powder, such as biscuits and cornbread.

	Cal	Fat g	Sat g	Chol mg
BREADS				
French hard roll (1)	124	0	0	0
White bread (1 sl)	67	1	0	1
Hot roll (1)	107	2	1	2
Buttered garlic bread (1 sl)	138	5	1	0
Cornbread (3″ × 3″ × 1″)	192	7	3	29
(See also Baked Goods, page 11, and Breads and Rolls, page 30)				
SPREADS				
Margarine (1 pat = 1 tsp)	34	4	1	0
Butter (1 pat = 1 tsp)	34	4	2	10
CRACKERS				
Melba toast (2)	38	0	0	0
Saltines (4)	52	2	0	0
Snack crackers (4)	60	3	1	0

c = cup; Cal = calories; Chol = cholesterol; diam = diameter; fl oz = fluid ounce; g = gram; lg = large; mayo = mayonnaise; med = medium; mg = milligram; na = not available; oz = ounce; prep = prepared; Sat = saturated fat; sl = slice; sm = small; Tbsp = tablespoon; tr = trace; tsp = teaspoon; w/ = with; w/o = without

---

**TIPS ON ORDERING
LOWER-FAT DESSERTS**

- Either skip dessert, split a serving with your dinner companion, or select fruit, angel food cake, sherbet, frozen yogurt, or gelatin (without sour cream, cream cheese, or whipped topping) instead of pie, cake, cookies, mousse, cheesecake, or ice cream. Most of the fat in fruit pie and cobbler is in the crust—reduce the fat by eating the filling and only a small amount of the crust. Most whipped toppings are high in fat and saturated fat, even those labeled "nondairy."
- Eat cake without frosting.

TIP ON LOWERING SODIUM

- Select fruit, gelatin, frozen yogurt, or sherbet instead of a baked dessert.

	Cal	Fat g	Sat g	Chol mg
Whole strawberries (6)	27	0	0	0
Wedge of honeydew (⅛ of melon)	56	0	0	0
Gelatin, plain (½ c)	80	0	0	0
w/whipped topping	110	2	2	0
Cakes				
Angel food (1/14 of cake)	137	0	0	0
Strawberry shortcake w/whipped topping	137	5	3	40
Pound (1/24 of 10" tube)	243	12	3	45
Pineapple upside down (3" × 3" × 2" high)	360	14	4	56
Applesauce w/cream cheese frosting (1/10 of 9" 2-layer cake)	628	27	12	118
Carrot w/cream cheese frosting (1/10 of 9" 2-layer cake)	628	27	12	118

	Cal	Fat g	Sat g	Chol mg
Chocolate w/chocolate butter cream frosting (1/10 of 9" 2-layer cake)	685	29	12	77
Fudge w/mocha frosting (1/10 of 9" 2-layer cake)	685	29	12	77
Frozen yogurt, low-fat (½ c)	87	1	1	4
Sherbet (½ c)	132	2	1	5
Pies (1/8 of 9" pie)				
Strawberry w/glaze, no whipped topping	210	9	3	5
w/whipped topping	449	28	20	5
Banana cream	269	12	5	65
Coconut cream	272	14	6	95
Lemon meringue	347	15	5	85
Cherry	345	17	7	10
Apple	381	20	7	10
Chocolate cream w/whipped topping	367	24	12	66
Ice Cream (½ c)	178	12	7	45
Sundae w/fudge sauce, nuts & whipped cream	351	19	11	109
Crêpes w/cherry filling (2)	283	15	8	135
Cheesecake (1/12 of 10" diam × 1½" high)	649	45	25	204

c = cup; Cal = calories; Chol = cholesterol; diam = diameter; fl oz = fluid ounce; g = gram; lg = large; mayo = mayonnaise; med = medium; mg = milligram; na = not available; oz = ounce; prep = prepared; Sat = saturated fat; sl = slice; sm = small; Tbsp = tablespoon; tr = trace; tsp = teaspoon; w/ = with; w/o = without

BEVERAGES

Americans consume a wide variety of beverages throughout the day and evening. This section contains information on choosing low-fat beverages and includes recommendations for alcohol consumption.

TIPS ON ORDERING BEVERAGES

- Ask for water if it is not provided.
- Choose milk that is skim, ½%, or 1% low-fat.
- Sparkling water, seltzer, and sugar-free soft drinks are refreshing while providing no calories. (Regular soft drinks have calories from sugar and other sweeteners.)
- Drink calorie-free beverages before and during the meal to reduce your hunger and help you feel satisfied.

	Cal	Fat g	Sat g	Chol mg
CARBONATED DRINKS (12 fl oz)				
Club soda	0	0	0	0
Diet cola	2	0	0	0
Ginger ale	124	0	0	0
Cola	151	0	0	0
Orange soda	177	0	0	0
COFFEE (6 fl oz)				
Black	4	0	0	0
w/1 Tbsp half & half	24	2	1	6
w/1 Tbsp powdered creamer	26	2	2	0
Cappuccino prep w/whole milk	64	3	2	14
FRUIT DRINKS (8 fl oz)				
Cranberry juice cocktail	108	0	0	0
Fruit punch	112	0	0	0
Grape drink	112	0	0	0
Citrus fruit juice	114	0	0	0
MILK AND MILK-BASED DRINKS				
Milk (8 fl oz)				
Skim	86	0	0	4
½% fat	92	1	1	7
1% fat	102	3	2	10
2% fat	121	5	3	18
Whole	150	8	5	33
Chocolate	208	8	5	30
Cocoa (1 pkg mix) prep w/water	120	3	2	130
Chocolate milkshake (10 fl oz)	360	11	7	37
Eggnog w/o alcohol (8 fl oz)	342	19	11	149
TEA (8 fl oz)				
Brewed or instant, plain	2	0	0	0
Instant w/sugar	87	0	0	0

c = cup; Cal = calories; Chol = cholesterol; diam = diameter; fl oz = fluid ounce; g = gram; lg = large; mayo = mayonnaise; med = medium; mg = milligram; na = not available; oz = ounce; prep = prepared; Sat = saturated fat; sl = slice; sm = small; Tbsp = tablespoon; tr = trace; tsp = teaspoon; w/ = with; w/o = without

Alcoholic beverages are high in calories, can increase your appetite, and tend to decrease your willpower. Health experts recommend limiting alcohol consumption to a maximum of two drinks per day.

ONE DRINK IS DEFINED AS:
- **1½ fluid ounces (fl oz) of distilled spirits, such as bourbon, rum, gin, scotch, etc.**
- **4 fl oz of table wine**
- **12 fl oz of regular beer**

Most common alcoholic drinks do not contain fat; however, fat is added to some mixed drinks in the form of cream, eggs, whole milk, or cream of coconut, and a few bottled alcoholic drinks contain cream. The first part of the following table provides the calories and grams of alcohol in selected alcoholic beverages (listed alphabetically), most of which contain no fat; those drinks containing fat, saturated fat, and/or cholesterol are listed in the second part of the table.

	Cal	Alcohol g
ALCOHOLIC BEVERAGES WITHOUT FAT		
Beer (12 fl oz)	148	13
Lite	101	12
"Near" beer	65	1
Black Russian (2¼ fl oz)	159	16
Bloody Mary (8 fl oz)	160	19
Bourbon and soda (4 fl oz)	97	14
Brandy Alexander (4 fl oz)	276	16
Champagne (6 fl oz)	124	16
Daiquiri, frozen (4 fl oz)	62	5
Not frozen (4 fl oz)	246	32

	Cal	Alcohol g
Gin, rum, vodka, whiskey (1½ fl oz)		
80 proof	97	14
86 proof	105	15
90 proof	110	16
94 proof	116	17
100 proof	124	18
Grasshopper (4 fl oz)	303	12
Hot buttered rum (4 fl oz)	145	13
Irish coffee (8 fl oz)	132	15
Long Island iced tea (4 fl oz)	111	11
Manhattan (4 fl oz)	216	30
Margarita w/crushed ice, frozen (12 fl oz)	185	16
Martini (4 fl oz)	222	32
Piña colada (12 fl oz)	618	14
Rum (see Gin)		
Rum and cola (4 fl oz)	91	8
Rum punch (4 fl oz)	128	14
Scotch and soda (4 fl oz)	97	14
Screwdriver (8 fl oz)	212	19
Vodka (see Gin)		
Vodka Collins (4 fl oz)	74	9
Vodka tonic (12 fl oz)	231	19
Whiskey (see Gin)		
White Russian (4 fl oz)	271	22
Wine		
Dessert or sweet (2 fl oz)	92	9
Red or white (6 fl oz)	124	16

	Cal	Fat g	Sat g	Chol mg
ALCOHOLIC BEVERAGES WITH FAT				
Brandy Alexander (4 fl oz)	276	8	5	26
Grasshopper (4 fl oz)	303	7	4	23
Hot buttered rum (4 fl oz)	145	6	3	14
Piña colada (12 fl oz)	618	29	25	0

c = cup; Cal = calories; Chol = cholesterol; diam = diameter; fl oz = fluid ounce; g = gram; lg = large; mayo = mayonnaise; med = medium; mg = milligram; na = not available; oz = ounce; prep = prepared; Sat = saturated fat; sl = slice; sm = small; Tbsp = tablespoon; tr = trace; tsp = teaspoon; w/ = with; w/o = without

SNACKS

Eating away from home can include snacks as well as meals. For some people, food eaten as snacks makes up a significant amount of the calories, fat, saturated fat, and cholesterol consumed each day. Snacking ranges from eating ice cream at a specialty shop, popcorn at a movie theater, and peanuts at a ball game to buying pretzels and a soft drink or picking up a candy bar for quick energy.

The following table gives you an idea of the calories, fat, saturated fat, and cholesterol content of selected snack foods. You can also find foods consumed as snacks in the Fast Food Section, starting on page 94. You will need to adjust these values if the snacks you eat differ in size from those listed below. Foods are arranged from low to high fat. Usually foods lower in fat are also lower in calories and saturated fat.

	Cal	Fat g	Sat g	Chol mg
SNACKS				
Frozen gelatin pop (1)	31	0	0	0
Frozen fruit & juice bar (3 fl oz)	75	0	0	0
Jelly beans (26 = 1 oz)	104	0	0	0
Hard candies (5 = 1 oz)	106	0	0	0
Gumdrops (20 = 1 oz)	109	0	0	0
Pretzels, hard (16 sm = 1 oz)	110	1	0	0
Popcorn or rice cakes (3)	114	1	0	0
Fruit leathers (1 oz)	97	2	0	0
Caramels (3½ = 1 oz)	109	2	2	4
Ice milk, soft serve, vanilla (½ cup = 3 oz)	111	2	1	10
Beef jerky (1 oz)	96	4	2	32
Frozen yogurt, soft serve, vanilla (½ cup = 2½ oz)	114	4	2	2
Pudding, ready-to-eat (5 oz)				
Lemon	177	4	1	0
Vanilla	185	5	1	10
Chocolate	189	6	1	5

	Cal	Fat g	Sat g	Chol mg
Granola bars (1 = 1 oz)				
Hard, chocolate chip	124	5	3	0
Hard, plain	134	6	1	0
Soft, chocolate chip coated w/milk chocolate	132	7	4	1
Hard, peanut butter	137	7	1	0
Tortilla chips (14 = 1 oz)	133	6	1	0
Cookies/Bars				
Oatmeal (3" diam × ¼" thick)	150	7	2	8
Sugar (3" diam × ¼" thick)	151	8	5	28
Chocolate chip (3" diam × ¼" thick)	155	9	4	23
Peanut butter (3" diam × ¼" thick)	161	9	2	9
Brownie w/nuts & frosting (3" × 3" × ½")	248	14	5	38
Popcorn (3 cups)				
Oil-popped	165	9	2	0
Caramel-coated w/peanuts	513	10	1	0
Popcorn w/"butter"	382	34	6	0
Milk-chocolate-coated peanuts (7 = 1 oz)	147	10	4	3
Banana chips (1 oz)	147	10	8	0
Potato chips, plain (14 = 1 oz)	152	10	3	0
Corn chips (14 = 1 oz)	153	10	1	0
Ice cream				
Soft serve, French vanilla (½ cup = 3 oz)	185	11	6	78
1 dip ice cream	178	12	7	45
Milk chocolate candy				
Plain (1½ oz = 1 bar)	225	13	8	10
w/almonds (14 pieces = 1½ oz)	239	18	5	0
Pork rind or skins, plain (2 oz = 1 bag)	311	18	6	54
Trail mix (½ c)				
Nuts, dried fruit & candy	346	22	4	0

c = cup; Cal = calories; Chol = cholesterol; diam = diameter; fl oz = fluid ounce; g = gram; lg = large; mayo = mayonnaise; med = medium; mg = milligram; na = not available; oz = ounce; prep = prepared; Sat = saturated fat; sl = slice; sm = small; Tbsp = tablespoon; tr = trace; tsp = teaspoon; w/ = with; w/o = without

Chapter 3

Ethnic Cuisines

Cuisines from a variety of different cultures are very popular in the United States. A National Restaurant Association survey showed that the three most popular ethnic cuisines in the United States are Chinese, Italian, and Mexican; of the people surveyed, 78% had tried Chinese food, 76% had tried Italian food, and 74% had tried Mexican food at some time.

Many ethnic cuisines are based on eating patterns that are naturally low in fat and calories. However, the Americanized versions of these foreign dishes are often higher in fat, saturated fat, cholesterol, and calories than the original foods, since they contain increased amounts of meat, cheese, and fat and smaller portions of grains, legumes, and vegetables. It is estimated that almost one third of the entrées ordered in the United States have foreign origins.

When eating in any type of restaurant, you may find it difficult to identify the foods lowest in fat, saturated fat, and cholesterol. This can be a greater challenge in ethnic restaurants, because you may not be familiar with some of the foods served; dishes may contain unknown ingredients and be prepared using unfamiliar techniques. This book includes information on 10 ethnic cuisines served in the United States. We visited chefs and restaurant owners and then analyzed recipes from cookbooks representing each cuisine; the resulting estimated calories and values for fat, saturated fat, and cholesterol, plus a brief description of each dish, appear on the following pages. The tables contain both dishes that are low in fat and those that are higher in fat. Although these values are estimates, you can use them to plan a total day's intake that will not exceed your recommended grams of fat (see page 151). We have listed the ethnic cuisines in this book in alphabetical order—from Cajun to Vietnamese.

CAJUN CUISINE

Southern Louisiana is famous for its Cajun food, a spicy cuisine that traces its roots back to southern France. Cajun foods such as seafood gumbo and blackened redfish are found on menus throughout the country. Roux is an ingredient unique to Cajun cooking; this cooked mixture of fat (animal fat or vegetable oil) and flour contributes to the high fat content of the gumbos, étouffées, sauces, and gravies typical of Cajun cooking. Shrimp, crayfish, and other seafood, which are often fried, are commonly featured as appetizers and entrées in Cajun cuisine. ''Blackened'' seafood is dipped in melted butter or oil and spices and cooked in a very hot skillet; chicken and beef can also be served blackened. Many Cajun dishes, such as red beans and rice, are served with sausage.

MENU TERMS THAT INDICATE HIGH FAT

Dirty rice—Prepared with chicken gizzards, chicken livers, ground pork, and butter or other fat

Gumbo, étouffée, sauces, and gravies made with roux (see description of roux above)

Hush puppies—Deep-fried cornmeal batter

TIPS ON ORDERING LOWER-FAT CAJUN FOOD

- Order boiled and grilled seafood rather than fried seafood as an appetizer or an entrée. Ask that blackened entrées be prepared with as little fat as possible. Shrimp and crayfish are low in fat (if not fried) but high in cholesterol.
- Request that sauces and gravies be served on the side or omitted.

Tips on Ordering Lower-Fat Cajun Food
(*continued*)

- Creole and jambalaya dishes may be lower in fat than gumbo and étouffée, depending on how they are prepared.
- Request white rice, even if it is seasoned with oil or margarine, as a substitute for "dirty" rice.
- Select menu items that do not include sausage. Order red beans and rice without the sausage commonly served as an accompaniment.

TIPS ON LOWERING SODIUM

- Select boiled seafood as an appetizer.
- Order grilled seafood, chicken, or steak as an entrée and request that it be prepared without salt.
- The sodium in gumbo, étouffée, jambalaya, and creole dishes cannot be reduced, since these dishes are prepared ahead of time.

The following table gives you an idea of the calories, fat, saturated fat, and cholesterol content of selected foods from Cajun cuisine. Whenever possible, several recipes were averaged to obtain the values listed; however, these figures are only estimates, and the content of an actual dish may vary, depending on how the chef prepares it. Within each section—appetizers, entrées, accompaniments, breads, and desserts—foods are arranged from low to high fat. Usually foods lower in fat are also lower in calories and saturated fat. If you do not see some of the lower-fat foods listed below on a restaurant menu, you may wish to request them.

	Cal	Fat g	Sat g	Chol mg
APPETIZERS				
Boiled Shrimp (12 extra lg)	103	1	0	203
Boiled Crayfish (12)	205	2	0	320
Oysters on the Half Shell (12)	121	4	1	97
SOUP				

Seafood Gumbo w/Sausage
   Roux-based soup w/seafood &
   sausage, served w/rice
	523	32	8	138

ENTRÉES				

Shrimp Creole
   Shrimp w/spicy tomato sauce,
   served w/rice
	385	13	6	170

Shrimp Jambalaya
   Highly seasoned rice dish
   w/tomatoes & shrimp
	423	16	5	185

Chicken Creole
   Chicken w/spicy tomato sauce,
   served w/rice
	640	24	6	98

Chicken & Seafood Jambalaya
   Highly seasoned rice dish
   w/tomatoes, chicken, &
   seafood
	839	24	7	168

Fried Shrimp (6–8)	454	25	5	201
Red Beans & Rice w/Ham Hocks & Sausage	865	35	13	78

Shrimp Étouffée
   Roux-based sauce w/shrimp,
   served w/rice
	619	39	18	227

Fried Catfish (8 oz)	729	39	7	116
ACCOMPANIMENTS				
Rice (¾ c)				
Seasoned w/margarine	246	3	1	0
Seasoned w/butter	246	3	2	6
Red Beans (¾ c)				
Seasoned w/ham hocks	147	5	2	14
Candied Yams (¾ c)				
w/butter & brown sugar sauce	341	9	5	23

	Cal	Fat g	Sat g	Chol mg
Dirty Rice				
Rice w/chicken gizzards, chicken livers, ground pork & butter	309	14	6	212
Corn Maque Choux (½ c)				
Corn w/milk, eggs, butter, margarine & oil	274	16	6	57
Kielbasa Sausage (4″ piece)	209	19	7	39

BREADS

	Cal	Fat g	Sat g	Chol mg
Cornbread (3″ × 3″ × 1″)	192	7	3	29
Hushpuppy (1)				
Deep-fried cornmeal batter	146	11	3	18

DESSERTS

	Cal	Fat g	Sat g	Chol mg
Pecan Praline (1)				
Candy made w/butter, sugar, cream & pecans	155	11	4	15
Bread Pudding (½ c) w/Lemon Sauce (3 Tbsp)				
Made w/bread, eggs, milk, butter & raisins	357	14	8	92

c = cup; Cal = calories; Chol = cholesterol; diam = diameter; fl oz = fluid ounce; g = gram; lg = large; mayo = mayonnaise; med = medium; mg = milligram; na = not available; oz = ounce; prep = prepared; Sat = saturated fat; sl = slice; sm = small; Tbsp = tablespoon; tr = trace; tsp = teaspoon; w/ = with; w/o = without

CHINESE CUISINE

Chinese food differs widely in flavor and fat content, depending on the region of China where the dish originated. The dishes most Americans think of as Chinese come from the south (Canton) and are steamed or stir-fried. Szechwan or Hunan foods, from western and central China, may be higher in fat and tend to be spicy from the chili peppers in them. Although rice is the staple in the eastern and coastal regions (Shanghai), food from the north and northeast (Beijing/Peking) is likely to be served with dumplings. Items such as fried egg rolls and fried butterfly shrimp with sweet-and-sour sauce, which are high in fat, are basic fare in Chinese restaurants; however, they are not part of typical Chinese meals and were actually developed in the United States.

MENU TERMS THAT INDICATE HIGH FAT

Crispy or fried—Food has been fried and is high in fat

Entrées with cashews or peanuts—Nuts often are deep-fried before being added to food

Sweet-and-sour entrées—Pork, shrimp, or chicken deep-fried, then stir-fried with vegetables in more oil before the addition of sweet-and-sour sauce

---

TIPS ON ORDERING LOWER-FAT CHINESE FOOD

- Since most Chinese dishes are prepared as they are ordered, special requests can usually be managed; ask that less oil be used to stir-fry.

Tips on Ordering Lower-Fat Chinese Food
(*continued*)

- Order fewer entrées than the number of people eating the meal; it is common practice for diners to share the generous portions served in many Chinese restaurants.
- Select steamed dumplings rather than egg rolls as an appetizer.
- Select dishes with lots of vegetables, such as chop suey with steamed rice.
- Steamed foods with a variety of sauces are better choices than fried items at dim sum lunches, which offer a variety of small appetizers.
- Eat the steamed rice served with most entrées instead of ordering fried rice.
- Order dishes with water chestnuts, which are fat-free, rather than with cashews and peanuts, which add fat.

TIPS ON LOWERING SODIUM

- Select steamed foods, such as dumplings or fish, and add sweet-and-sour sauce at the table.
- Ask that MSG (monosodium glutamate) not be used in food. MSG cannot be left out of commercially prepared sauces.
- Select entrées not prepared with oyster or bean sauce, which are high in sodium.
- Soy sauce, which is very high in sodium, is often used in stir-fried dishes; ask that it be omitted.
- Use sweet-and-sour sauce, plum sauce, or duck sauce instead of soy sauce at the table.

The following table gives you an idea of the calories, fat, saturated fat, and cholesterol content of selected foods from Chinese cuisine. Whenever possible, several recipes were averaged to obtain the values listed; however, these figures are only estimates, and the content of an actual dish may vary, depending on how the chef prepares it. Within each section—appetizers, soups, entrées, accompaniments, sauces, and desserts—foods are arranged from low to high fat. Usually foods lower in fat are also lower in calories and saturated fat. If you do not see some of the lower-fat foods listed below on a restaurant menu, you may wish to request them.

	Cal	Fat g	Sat g	Chol mg
APPETIZERS				
Steamed Vegetable Dumplings (6)	288	5	1	51
Spring Roll, fried (1 lg)	176	15	3	8
Egg Rolls (2 lg)	263	17	5	79
Fried Won Ton (6)	408	18	6	144
Fried Beef or Pork Dumplings (6)	517	26	7	94
Fried Chicken Wings (6)	558	40	10	90
Shrimp Toast (4 sm pieces)	505	46	9	54
SOUPS				
Egg Drop (1 c)	103	4	1	106
Velvet Corn (1 c)	172	5	1	106
Won Ton (1 c w/4 or 5 won tons)	326	9	3	60
Hot & Sour (1 c)	226	12	3	83
ENTRÉES				
Chop Suey (1½ c) w/steamed rice (1½ c)				
w/vegetables	586	10	3	0
w/chicken & shrimp	614	10	3	74
w/beef & pork	709	21	7	45
Szechuan-Style Eggplant	145	11	2	0
Pepper Steak	225	12	4	56
Shrimp w/Snow Peas (2 c)	239	12	2	133
Eggplant & Peppers	187	14	2	0
Shredded Pork w/Garlic or Peking Sauce	212	14	4	51
Snow Peas w/Water Chestnuts (2 c)	214	14	2	0

	Cal	Fat g	Sat g	Chol mg
Peas & Sausage	198	15	4	33
Hunan Chicken Cold shredded chicken	274	15	3	74
Shredded Beef w/Green Peppers	239	17	4	43
Shrimp w/Cashews	235	19	3	53
Beef & Broccoli	233	20	4	29
Pork in Hoisin Sauce	315	21	8	70
Moo Goo Gai Pan Chicken stir-fried w/vegetables	380	24	4	62
Sweet-and-Sour Meat Breaded & fried cubes of meat w/sweet-and-sour sauce				
w/shrimp	565	25	4	215
w/chicken	625	27	5	83
w/pork	735	37	8	95
Chow Mein (1½ c) w/crisp chow mein noodles (1½ c)				
w/vegetables	545	30	5	0
w/chicken & shrimp	573	30	5	74
w/beef & pork	668	41	10	45
Beef w/Asparagus	360	31	6	43
Mongolian Beef Stir-fried beef & green onions over fried rice noodles	503	34	7	86
Lemon Chicken Breaded & fried chicken w/lemon sauce	784	35	6	124
Fried Bean Curd	519	39	6	53

ACCOMPANIMENTS

	Cal	Fat g	Sat g	Chol mg
Steamed White Rice (1 c)	241	0	0	0
Fried Rice (1 c) Cooked rice fried in oil	370	13	3	128

SAUCES

	Cal	Fat g	Sat g	Chol mg
Worcestershire Sauce (1 Tbsp)	10	0	0	0
Sweet-and-Sour Sauce (1 Tbsp)	18	0	0	0

c = cup; Cal = calories; Chol = cholesterol; diam = diameter; fl oz = fluid ounce; g = gram; lg = large; mayo = mayonnaise; med = medium; mg = milligram; na = not available; oz = ounce; prep = prepared; Sat = saturated fat; sl = slice; sm = small; Tbsp = tablespoon; tr = trace; tsp = teaspoon; w/ = with; w/o = without

	Cal	Fat g	Sat g	Chol mg
Sauces *(continued)*				
Plum or Duck Sauce (1 Tbsp)	26	2	0	0
Sesame Soy Dip (1 Tbsp)	31	2	0	0
Mustard Sauce (1 Tbsp)	31	3	0	0
Hot Chili Sauce (1 Tbsp)	86	8	1	0

DESSERTS

	Cal	Fat g	Sat g	Chol mg
Fortune Cookie (1)	29	0	0	1
Lychee (½ c)				
Fruit in syrup	57	0	0	0
Bean Curd w/Soybean Milk	435	30	5	29

c = cup; Cal = calories; Chol = cholesterol; diam = diameter; fl oz = fluid ounce; g = gram; lg = large; mayo = mayonnaise; med = medium; mg = milligram; na = not available; oz = ounce; prep = prepared; Sat = saturated fat; sl = slice; sm = small; Tbsp = tablespoon; tr = trace; tsp = teaspoon; w/ = with; w/o = without

FRENCH CUISINE

Classic French cuisine is known for its rich dishes, in which sauce with butter is often a key ingredient. In 1972 a new movement started that rejected overly rich, complicated dishes, not suitable for health-conscious individuals. Advocates of the "nouvelle cuisine" seek fresh ingredients, lighter dishes, and simpler cooking methods, including the use of lower-fat, lighter sauces based on meat juices, stocks, and spices. Rapid cooking without fat is often used in nouvelle cuisine. Foods offered by the "new cooks" include crisp vegetables, prepared to retain their natural flavors; thin-sliced meat with the fat trimmed off; airy mousses; vegetable purées; and light fruity sauces to accompany desserts. Most French restaurants offer a combination of nouvelle cuisine and traditional dishes.

MENU TERMS THAT INDICATE HIGH FAT

Au gratin—Foods that are topped with cheese and, sometimes, butter

Béarnaise—Classic sauce containing butter and egg yolk, which is served with grilled meat, fowl, and eggs

Béchamel—Basic white sauce of milk, flour, and butter

Crème fraîche—Tangy heavy cream

Hollandaise—Sauce made with butter, egg yolks, and lemon juice

Mornay—Béchamel sauce with additional butter, grated Parmesan and Gruyère cheeses, and, possibly, egg yolk

Pâté—Rich mixture or spread made of meat, poultry, game, fish, or vegetables; pâté de foie gras is a smooth rich pâté made with goose liver

---

TIPS ON ORDERING
LOWER-FAT FRENCH FOOD

- Choosing simple dishes is the best way to keep your meal low in fat while enjoying French cuisine.
- If you order a dish with an added sauce, ask that it be served in a side dish so that you can control the amount you use. Usually wine sauces, such as bordelaise, are lower in fat. Avoid the common practice of soaking up rich sauces with bread.
- Select French bread rather than croissants.
- Often chefs add butter to sauces immediately before serving, significantly increasing the fat in a dish such as Moules Marinières (see following table); request that the chef not add extra butter or oil prior to serving French dishes.
- For dessert, choose sorbet, which is a water ice containing beaten egg white and flavored with fruit juice or purée or other flavoring.

TIP ON LOWERING SODIUM

- Choose cooked-to-order dishes, such as grilled fish and vegetables, and ask that salt be omitted during preparation.

The following table gives you an idea of the calories, fat, saturated fat, and cholesterol content of selected foods from French cuisine. Whenever possible, several recipes were averaged to obtain the values listed; however, these figures are only estimates, and the content of an actual dish may vary, depending on how the chef prepares it. Within each section—appetizers, soups, salads, fish and meat entrées, breads, and desserts—foods are arranged from low to high fat. Usually foods lower in fat are also lower in calories and saturated fat. If you do not see some of the lower-fat foods listed below on a restaurant menu, you may wish to request them.

	Cal	Fat g	Sat g	Chol mg
HORS D'OEUVRES (APPETIZERS)				
Melon au Porto				
Cantaloupe w/port	231	1	0	0
Oysters on the Half Shell (6)	61	2	1	48
Moules Marinière				
Mussels steamed in wine w/shallots sautéed in butter	156	5	3	48
w/extra butter added to sauce before serving	289	20	12	96
Pâté de Campagne (1 sl)				
Coarse loaf made w/pork loin, liver & seasonings, served cold	283	16	6	203
Escargots à la Bourguignone				
Snails baked in their shells w/garlic butter (6)	251	24	14	82
POTAGES (SOUPS)				
Soupe à l'Oignon				
Onion soup w/Swiss cheese	309	13	7	33
Bisque de Homard				
Lobster bisque	252	16	9	75
Vichyssoise				
Chilled leek & potato cream soup	277	21	13	65
SALADES (SALADS)				
Panachée				
Mixed green salad	12	0	0	0
w/vinaigrette dressing	144	14	2	0
César (2 c)				
Caesar salad	167	15	3	46

c = cup; Cal = calories; Chol = cholesterol; diam = diameter; fl oz = fluid ounce; g = gram; lg = large; mayo = mayonnaise; med = medium; mg = milligram; na = not available; oz = ounce; prep = prepared; Sat = saturated fat; sl = slice; sm = small; Tbsp = tablespoon; tr = trace; tsp = teaspoon; w/ = with; w/o = without

	Cal	Fat g	Sat g	Chol mg
Salades (Salads) *(continued)*				
Niçoise				
Salad w/eggs, olives, tomatoes & anchovies (recipes vary greatly)	443	26	4	149

POISSONS (FISH)

	Cal	Fat g	Sat g	Chol mg
Grilled Tuna on Bed of Roasted Peppers w/Balsamic Vinegar Sauce (8 oz)	294	9	3	116
Salmon Fillet (8 oz) w/Smoked Salmon & Horseradish Crust	518	22	7	111
Homard au Beurre d'Herbes Lobster (sm) w/herb butter	322	24	14	147
Salmon Sautéed in Butter (8 oz) w/zucchini "noodles" & red pepper purée	593	32	13	141
Truite Amandine (8 oz) Sautéed trout w/almonds in butter sauce	668	51	24	179
Fillet de Sole Meunière (8 oz) Sautéed sole in butter sauce	751	60	36	260

VIANDES ET VOLAILLES (MEAT AND POULTRY)

	Cal	Fat g	Sat g	Chol mg
Magret de Canard (6 oz) Breast of duck browned in goose fat, w/o skin	277	15	6	117
w/skin	545	47	16	131
Gigot d'Agneau (8 oz) Leg of lamb (trimmed)	347	16	6	156
Paupiette de Veau Braisée (1) Rolled veal stuffed w/ground pork & sautéed in butter	292	18	8	115
Rognons d'Agneau Grillés (4 oz) Lamb kidney w/bacon, basted w/butter	321	19	7	661
Coq au Vin (6 oz) Chicken stew w/wine, onion, mushrooms & bacon, chicken w/o skin	541	20	6	121
w/skin	664	31	9	150

	Cal	Fat g	Sat g	Chol mg
Steak au Poivre (8 oz)				
Steak w/crushed peppercorns, trimmed, pan-fried in butter & served w/o drippings	436	22	10	158
Côtes d'Agneau Grillées (2)				
Broiled lamb chops (trimmed)	395	25	8	137
Boeuf Bourguignon				
Beef stew w/Burgundy, onions, mushrooms & bacon	801	31	11	240
Rôti de Porc (6 oz)				
Roast loin of pork (trimmed)	571	32	11	204
Lapin en Gibelotte				
Rabbit stew w/wine	630	32	11	178
PAINS (BREADS)				
French Bread (1 med roll)	156	1	0	1
Croissant (1 med)	232	12	7	50
DESSERTS				
Sorbet (½ c)	125	0	0	0
Crêpe Suzette (1)				
Thin pancake in orange butter sauce, flavored w/orange liqueur & flamed	205	11	7	56
Crème Caramel (¾ c)				
Caramelized custard	348	11	5	270
Banane Flambée (1)				
Flamed banana	328	16	10	41
Tarte aux Pommes (1/10 of 9" diam)				
Open-face apple pie	305	17	10	43
Mousse au Chocolat (¾ c)				
Chocolate mousse	303	25	14	194

c = cup; Cal = calories; Chol = cholesterol; diam = diameter; fl oz = fluid ounce; g = gram; lg = large; mayo = mayonnaise; med = medium; mg = milligram; na = not available; oz = ounce; prep = prepared; Sat = saturated fat; sl = slice; sm = small; Tbsp = tablespoon; tr = trace; tsp = teaspoon; w/ = with; w/o = without

GREEK AND MIDDLE EASTERN CUISINE

The cuisines of Greece and Middle Eastern countries, such as Lebanon, share a number of common dishes. Many Greek and Middle Eastern dishes are high in fat because of the lavish use of oil, usually olive oil. Popular grain dishes include rice pilaf, couscous, and tabouli, which typically contain olive oil. Chickpeas are often puréed with fava beans to make falafel or mashed with sesame seed paste (tahini) to make hummus.

MENU TERMS THAT INDICATE HIGH FAT

Baklava—Sweet dessert made of phyllo dough, honey, butter, and nuts

Falafel—Deep-fried ball or patty of minced chickpeas and/or fava beans

Feta—White medium-fat goat's- or ewe's-milk cheese; when made outside Greece, it may be made from cow's milk or a combination of cow's and goat's milk

Hummus—Flavored mashed chickpeas with tahini and, usually, olive oil

Loukanika—Sausage

Tahini—Seasoned paste of crushed raw sesame seeds, used in many dishes

---

TIPS ON ORDERING LOWER-FAT GREEK AND MIDDLE EASTERN FOODS

- As an appetizer, select baked stuffed eggplant, rice mixtures wrapped in grape leaves, or cucumber and yogurt dip rather than fried calamari (squid), fish roe dip, or hummus.
- Ask that the olive oil often added to the top of dips, such as hummus and fish roe dip, and other prepared dishes be omitted.
- When ordering Greek salad, ask that the feta cheese and olives be served on the side so you can control the amount eaten.

Tips on Ordering Lower-Fat Greek and Middle Eastern Foods (*continued*)

- Pita bread, which is often served with appetizers and entrées, is low in fat.
- Choose a chicken pita sandwich instead of a gyro, which contains beef and lamb; yogurt-cucumber sauce can be served on the side so that you can control the amount eaten.
- Since casseroles are made ahead of time, there is no way the fat in them can be reduced. Some restaurants offer small portions of several typical Greek and Middle Eastern foods on a combination plate which can be shared with a dinner companion.
- When you order grilled fish or baked chicken, specify that only a small amount of olive oil be used in preparation and that none be "added"; often lavish amounts of olive oil are added to these dishes before they are served.
- Request that lean meat be used in a shish kabab and that butter not be used to baste it.
- Rizogalo (rice pudding) is lower in fat than baklava (pastry) or galatoboureko (custard pie). Split a dessert with your dinner companion.

TIPS ON LOWERING SODIUM

- Choose cooked-to-order dishes, such as baked fish, and ask that salt be omitted during food preparation.
- The sodium in casseroles, such as moussaka and spanakopita, dips, and sauces that are made ahead of time, cannot be reduced.
- Feta cheese is higher in sodium than cheddar; it contains about the same amount of sodium as many processed cheeses.

The following table gives you an idea of the calories, fat, saturated fat, and cholesterol content of selected foods from Greek and Middle Eastern cuisine. Whenever possible, several recipes were averaged to obtain the values listed; however, these figures are only estimates, and the content of an actual dish may vary, depending on how the chef prepares it. Within each section—appetizers, entrées, accompaniments, and desserts—foods are arranged from low to high fat. Usually foods lower in fat are also lower in calories and saturated fat. If you do not see some of the lower-fat foods listed below on a restaurant menu, you may wish to request them.

	Cal	Fat g	Sat g	Chol mg
APPETIZERS				
Yogurt & Cucumber Salad	115	7	3	13
Tzatziki (⅓ c)				
Yogurt & cucumber dip w/garlic & olive oil	107	8	3	12
Hummus (⅓ c)				
Puréed chickpea dip w/tahini & garlic	178	11	1	0
Spanakopita				
Spinach & cheese tart	182	14	6	43
Dolmades (8)				
Grape leaves stuffed w/rice & vegetables and/or fruits	254	14	2	0
Kota Soupa Avgolemono				
Chicken & rice soup w/egg & lemon	477	20	6	220
Taramosalata (⅓ c)				
Fish roe dip w/onion & olive oil	356	27	4	69
ENTRÉES				
Plaki				
Baked fish w/tomatoes, onions & olive oil	391	17	4	102
w/tomatoes, potatoes & olive oil	625	24	4	212

	Cal	Fat g	Sat g	Chol mg
Keftedes				
Meatballs (6–8 small or 25 tiny)	404	25	9	157
Souvlaki				
Shish kebab w/meat (4 oz) & vegetables	371	26	10	96
Dolmades Me Lahano (4)				
Cabbage leaves stuffed w/meat & rice w/egg & lemon sauce	457	26	9	166
Gyro Sandwich				
Beef & lamb (5 oz) in pita bread w/yogurt sauce	546	28	11	126
Dolmades (8)				
Grape leaves stuffed w/meat & rice w/egg & lemon sauce	465	29	10	193
Baked Lamb with Orzo				
Lamb (4½ oz) & pasta w/onion & tomato	603	31	14	123
Spanakopita				
Spinach pie w/egg & cheese	570	35	11	172
Moussaka				
Eggplant casserole w/ground meat	564	39	15	136
Pastitsio				
Baked macaroni & meat pie	784	44	23	248
Roast Leg of Lamb				
Lamb (7 oz) basted w/butter and/or olive oil, served w/roasted potatoes	1074	74	25	283

ACCOMPANIMENTS

	Cal	Fat g	Sat g	Chol mg
Pilaf				
Rice w/butter & seasonings	322	8	5	21
w/spinach	398	17	2	0
w/chicken	557	26	11	128
Baymes				
Baked okra	147	10	1	0

c = cup; Cal = calories; Chol = cholesterol; diam = diameter; fl oz = fluid ounce; g = gram; lg = large; mayo = mayonnaise; med = medium; mg = milligram; na = not available; oz = ounce; prep = prepared; Sat = saturated fat; sl = slice; sm = small; Tbsp = tablespoon; tr = trace; tsp = teaspoon; w/ = with; w/o = without

	Cal	Fat g	Sat g	Chol mg
Accompaniments *(continued)*				
Couscous				
Farina w/chicken stock & butter	215	17	5	16
w/meat, vegetables, olive oil & butter	681	38	11	114

BREADS

	Cal	Fat g	Sat g	Chol mg
Pita (1)				
Round flatbread	164	0	0	0

DESSERTS

	Cal	Fat g	Sat g	Chol mg
Rizogalo				
Creamy rice pudding	212	8	4	92
Baklava				
Pastry of phyllo, nuts, butter & syrup or honey	244	15	5	19
Tourta Mocha				
Mocha torte	373	17	11	150
Galatoboureko				
Custard pie w/phyllo pastry	524	21	11	118

c = cup; Cal = calories; Chol = cholesterol; diam = diameter; fl oz = fluid ounce; g = gram; lg = large; mayo = mayonnaise; med = medium; mg = milligram; na = not available; oz = ounce; prep = prepared; Sat = saturated fat; sl = slice; sm = small; Tbsp = tablespoon; tr = trace; tsp = teaspoon; w/ = with; w/o = without

INDIAN CUISINE

The imaginative use of spices is characteristic of foods originating in India. Some, but not all, Indian dishes are hot from the use of chili peppers. Spices are typically heated in oil; then vegetables, yogurt, cream, and/or meat are added. In Indian cooking, fat is often not drained off after meat or vegetables are cooked.

MENU TERMS THAT INDICATE HIGH FAT

Ghee—Clarified butter
Korma—Braised meat with rich yogurt and cream sauce
Malai—Heavy cream or cream sauce
Pakora—Deep-fried dough with vegetables

TIPS ON ORDERING LOWER-FAT INDIAN FOOD

- Select bread and meat cooked in a tandoor (special oven), and request that oil or ghee not be brushed on them.
- Choose a raita or vegetable salad, which is usually served with lemon juice.
- Select a kebab or tandoori entrée (not brushed with fat) instead of a dish with sauce, such as curry; sauces are prepared ahead of time and cannot be specially made with less fat.
- Choose tikka or tandoori meats, since both are low in fat when they are not brushed with fat.

TIP ON LOWERING SODIUM

- Select tandoori or tikka meat as an entrée; they are lower in sodium than entrées with sauce, such as curry.

The following table gives you an idea of the calories, fat, saturated fat, and cholesterol content of selected foods from Indian cuisine. Whenever possible, several recipes were averaged to obtain the values listed; however, these figures are only estimates, and the content of an actual dish may vary, depending on how the chef prepares it. Within each section—appetizers, entrées, accompaniments, breads, desserts, and beverages—foods are arranged from low to high fat. Usually foods lower in fat are also lower in calories and saturated fat. If you do not see some of the lower-fat foods listed below on a restaurant menu, you may wish to request them.

	Cal	Fat g	Sat g	Chol mg
APPETIZERS				
Tikkas Chicken Tandoori (1 thigh)				
Marinated chicken cooked in tandoori				
Not brushed w/fat	114	6	2	46
Brushed w/butter	182	13	6	67
Bhujias (2)				
Onion fritters	106	10	2	0
Gobhi Pakoras (2)				
Cauliflower fritters	196	10	2	0
Samosa (1)				
Deep-fried pastry filled w/chicken & peas	205	12	2	21
ENTRÉES				
Jhinga Tandoori (6–8 lg)				
Marinated shrimp cooked in tandoori				
Not brushed w/fat	77	2	0	123
Brushed w/butter	145	10	5	144
Tandoori Chicken (¼ chicken)				
Not brushed w/fat	249	11	3	102
Brushed w/butter after cooking	317	19	8	122
Chicken Chaat				
Cold shredded chicken w/spices on lettuce	329	11	4	119

	Cal	Fat g	Sat g	Chol mg
Murgh Reshmi Kabab (5 oz)				
Marinated chicken kebab				
Not brushed w/fat	271	12	3	111
Brushed w/butter	339	20	8	131
Machli Masala				
Fish curry	337	12	3	124
Gosht Vindaloo				
Beef or lamb w/potatoes in				
tangy sauce	266	19	9	79
Tandoori Lamb (8 oz)				
Not brushed w/fat	370	19	6	150
Brushed w/butter	438	27	11	171
Badam Korma				
Fried onions & mutton in yogurt				
sauce w/almonds	354	22	10	115
Jhinga Masala				
Shrimp in tomato cream sauce	307	24	8	136
Murgh Kari				
Chicken curry	483	28	8	131
Rogan Josh				
Lamb curry	440	29	7	99
Badsahi Badam Korma				
Lamb curry w/almonds	525	32	13	175
Nawabi Biryani				
Rice & lamb w/fat & spices	809	32	12	85
Murgh Makhani				
Butter chicken	626	45	25	220
Gosht Do Piaza				
Fried lamb & onions simmered				
in spices & juice	696	49	13	163

ACCOMPANIMENTS

	Cal	Fat g	Sat g	Chol mg
Katchumber Salad				
Cucumber, onion & tomato				
salad w/oil & lemon on				
lettuce leaf	69	3	0	0
Raita (⅔ c)				
Spiced yogurt w/cucumber	83	4	3	16

c = cup; Cal = calories; Chol = cholesterol; diam = diameter; fl oz = fluid ounce; g = gram; lg = large; mayo = mayonnaise; med = medium; mg = milligram; na = not available; oz = ounce; prep = prepared; Sat = saturated fat; sl = slice; sm = small; Tbsp = tablespoon; tr = trace; tsp = teaspoon; w/ = with; w/o = without

	Cal	Fat g	Sat g	Chol mg
Accompaniments *(continued)*				
Matar Pulao				
Rice pilaf w/peas	370	7	4	16
Gobhi Matar Tamatar				
Cauliflower w/peas & tomatoes	159	8	1	0
Navarattan Curry				
Nine-vegetable curry	225	12	7	33
Matar Paneer				
Fried cheese w/peas	362	21	8	44
Malai Kofta				
Creamed vegetable balls	334	22	10	43
Tarkari Biryani				
Rice w/vegetables	715	26	15	64
Dal Maharani				
Creamed lentils w/spices	471	27	14	64
Saag Paneer				
Spinach w/cheese cubes in				
cream sauce	564	35	16	92

BREADS

	Cal	Fat g	Sat g	Chol mg
Chapati or Roti (1)				
Bread cooked on griddle				
Not brushed w/oil	62	2	0	0
Brushed w/oil	102	7	1	0
Naan (1)				
Bread baked in tandoori				
Not brushed w/butter	188	10	5	112
Brushed w/butter	222	14	8	122
Paratha (1)				
Flaky wheat bread fried on				
griddle	226	14	8	36
Onion Kulcha (1)				
Naan stuffed w/onions & spices	256	16	9	129
Keema Paratha (1)				
Bread stuffed w/meat & buttered	267	17	10	48

DESSERTS

	Cal	Fat g	Sat g	Chol mg
Aam Malai				
Mango ice cream	268	13	8	103
Kheer				
Indian rice pudding	414	13	7	44

	Cal	Fat g	Sat g	Chol mg
Gulab Jamons				
Fried milk balls in rose water & sugar syrup	246	15	7	41
Rasomalai				
Dumplings w/whipped cream & pistachios	435	23	14	83
Kulfi				
Ice cream w/pistachios, almonds & rose essence	399	26	13	75

BEVERAGES

	Cal	Fat g	Sat g	Chol mg
Sweet Lassi	120	2	2	9
Whole-milk yogurt w/sugar & water				
Spiced Tea w/whole milk	89	3	2	12

c = cup; Cal = calories; Chol = cholesterol; diam = diameter; fl oz = fluid ounce; g = gram; lg = large; mayo = mayonnaise; med = medium; mg = milligram; na = not available; oz = ounce; prep = prepared; Sat = saturated fat; sl = slice; sm = small; Tbsp = tablespoon; tr = trace; tsp = teaspoon; w/ = with; w/o = without

ITALIAN CUISINE

Pasta is central to most dishes served in Italian restaurants. The richness of a pasta dish is determined by the type of sauce, amount of cheese, and type of meat in it. Italian cuisine in the United States is similar to dishes native to southern Italy, which use tomato sauces instead of the high-fat creamy sauces more common to northern Italian cuisine. Marinara sauce is a popular tomato-based sauce; although it usually is not low in fat because of the oil used in preparation, it is low in saturated fat. (For pizza, see page 32.)

MENU TERMS THAT INDICATE HIGH FAT

Alfredo—Sauce made with butter, cream, and cheese
Crema—Cream
Gelato—Italian ice cream
Parmigiana—Food is floured, fried, then baked with cheese

TIPS ON ORDERING LOWER-FAT ITALIAN FOOD

- Choose "cook-to-order" dishes and ask that the oil used be reduced; examples are meat, fish, poultry, or vegetables served with pasta.
- Select red sauces, such as pomodoro and marinara sauce, rather than cream sauces, such as Alfredo sauce.
- Casserole-type dishes (lasagne, ravioli, etc.) contain high-fat ingredients, such as ground meat, sausage, cheese, cream, and butter.
- If an entrée is served with fettuccine Alfredo, request that marinara sauce be substituted.

The following table gives you an idea of the
calories, fat, saturated fat, and cholesterol content
of selected foods from Italian cuisine. Whenever
possible, several recipes were averaged to obtain
the values listed; however, these figures are only
estimates, and the content of an actual dish may
vary, depending on how the chef prepares it.
Within each section—appetizers, entrées, accompaniments, and desserts—foods are arranged
from low to high fat. Usually foods lower in fat are
also lower in calories and saturated fat. If you do
not see some of the lower-fat foods listed below on
a restaurant menu, you may wish to request them.

	Cal	Fat g	Sat g	Chol mg
APPETIZERS				
Roasted Peppers				
Marinated in olive oil	45	3	0	0
w/olive oil & anchovies	63	3	1	9
Stracciatella (1½ c)				
Chicken broth w/egg, pasta &				
Parmesan cheese	160	6	3	115
Minestrone (1½ c)				
Vegetable soup w/beans	204	7	1	0
w/beans & meat	245	8	2	20
Tortellini in Brodo (1½ c)				
Pasta in broth	189	10	5	55
Caponata				
Sautéed eggplant w/olives,				
peppers, tomatoes & other				
vegetables	200	13	2	0

c = cup; Cal = calories; Chol = cholesterol; diam = diameter; fl oz
= fluid ounce; g = gram; lg = large; mayo = mayonnaise; med =
medium; mg = milligram; na = not available; oz = ounce; prep =
prepared; Sat = saturated fat; sl = slice; sm = small; Tbsp = tablespoon; tr = trace; tsp = teaspoon; w/ = with; w/o = without

	Cal	Fat g	Sat g	Chol mg
Appetizers *(continued)*				
Fried Calamari				
Breaded & fried squid	291	14	4	239
Stuffed Artichoke (1)	515	19	4	13

ENTRÉES

	Cal	Fat g	Sat g	Chol mg
Shrimp Scampi, marinated in oil & broiled	110	3	1	160
Sautéed in oil w/sauce	240	15	2	221
Linguine (1¾ c) w/Clam Sauce				
w/red sauce (¾ c)	575	12	2	33
w/white wine sauce (¾ c)	574	13	4	53
w/cream sauce (1¼ c)	760	39	23	132
Pasta Primavera				
Pasta w/sautéed vegetables & tomato sauce (1¾ c pasta w/⅔ c sauce)	520	14	2	0
Spaghetti w/Marinara Sauce				
Pasta w/tomato sauce (2 c spaghetti w/¾ c sauce)	585	15	3	4
Veal Marsala				
Breaded, fried & cooked w/wine	296	17	7	96
Veal Scaloppine				
Breaded & sautéed	337	19	8	143
Meatball & Tomato Sauce on a Submarine Roll	480	23	8	78
Chicken Marsala (2 or 3 pieces of chicken)				
Sautéed & cooked in wine sauce	440	25	7	140
Chicken Cacciatore (2 pieces of chicken)				
Sautéed & cooked w/wine, onion & tomato	532	29	8	152
Spaghetti & Meatballs in Tomato Sauce (2 c spaghetti & 4 med meatballs)	795	29	10	173
Veal Parmigiana				
Breaded, fried & baked w/cheese	514	32	14	138

	Cal	Fat g	Sat g	Chol mg
Spaghetti w/Italian Sausage & Marinara Sauce (2 c spaghetti w/7"-long Italian sausage)	791	32	11	77
Spaghetti w/Meat Sauce (1¾ c spaghetti w/1 c sauce)	804	35	13	79
Lasagne w/Meat				
Pasta baked w/meat sauce & cheese	697	36	15	145
w/meat sauce, cheese & white sauce	746	49	26	249
Fettuccine Alfredo (1¾ c pasta w/½ c sauce)				
Pasta w/sauce of butter, cream & Parmesan cheese	697	40	23	197
Cannelloni (2, each 6" long)				
Tube pasta stuffed w/meat, cheese & sautéed vegetables & covered w/sauce	808	59	27	368
Eggplant Parmesan				
Breaded, fried & baked w/cheese	1051	98	21	66

ACCOMPANIMENTS

	Cal	Fat g	Sat g	Chol mg
Risotto				
Rice w/butter & chicken stock (1 c)	159	3	1	5
w/wine & cheese (1½ c)	420	12	7	30
w/wine & fruit (1½ c)	505	16	9	45
w/vegetables & cheese (1½ c)	474	17	9	39
Polenta (1 c)				
Cornmeal pudding (eaten in place of pasta or bread)	172	4	2	10
Italian Spinach				
Fresh spinach sautéed in oil	114	10	1	0
w/bacon & Parmesan cheese	142	9	3	8
w/pine nuts & raisins	196	16	6	22
w/ham, pine nuts & raisins	287	21	7	33

c = cup; Cal = calories; Chol = cholesterol; diam = diameter; fl oz = fluid ounce; g = gram; lg = large; mayo = mayonnaise; med = medium; mg = milligram; na = not available; oz = ounce; prep = prepared; Sat = saturated fat; sl = slice; sm = small; Tbsp = tablespoon; tr = trace; tsp = teaspoon; w/ = with; w/o = without

	Cal	Fat g	Sat g	Chol mg
DESSERTS				
Coffee Granita (½ c)				
Coffee ice	159	0	0	0
w/whipped cream	151	11	7	40
Zabaglione (hot or cold)				
Frothy mixture of egg yolk, sugar & wine	135	5	1	195
w/cream & fruit	294	21	11	284
w/cream & other flavorings	328	20	12	202
Tira Mi Su				
Mixture of coffee, cookies, mascarpone or cream cheese, egg yolk, rum or brandy & cocoa	383	25	15	206
BEVERAGES				
Cappuccino				
Espresso coffee & milk (1 c)	80	3	2	0

c = cup; Cal = calories; Chol = cholesterol; diam = diameter; fl oz = fluid ounce; g = gram; lg = large; mayo = mayonnaise; med = medium; mg = milligram; na = not available; oz = ounce; prep = prepared; Sat = saturated fat; sl = slice; sm = small; Tbsp = tablespoon; tr = trace; tsp = teaspoon; w/ = with; w/o = without

JAPANESE CUISINE

Many of the selections available in Japanese restaurants are low in fat and saturated fat. Japanese dishes typically contain a lot of rice and vegetables, small amounts of meat, fish, and poultry, and little added fat. Seafood, which is very low in fat and saturated fat, is very important in Japanese cuisine. Many Japanese restaurants flamboyantly prepare food right in front of you.

MENU TERMS THAT INDICATE HIGH FAT

Agedashi—Fried tofu
Tempura—Seafood and/or vegetables dipped in batter and deep-fried
Tonkatsu—Breaded and fried pork cutlet

TIPS ON ORDERING LOWER-FAT JAPANESE FOOD

- Most Japanese sauces do not contain fat, and foods are typically not stir-fried.
- Sashimi (sliced raw fish) and sushi (vinegared rice with seafood that is usually raw) are low in fat; sushi may also contain a small egg omelet, vegetables, or avocado. (Note: Raw fish can contain parasites, bacteria, and viruses.)
- Select clear soups, such as sumashi wan, which are usually low in fat; some clear soups may contain added egg.
- Choose low-fat entrées, such as yosenabe, teriyaki, shabu shabu, and sukiyaki.
- Some noodle dishes, such as su udon, are low in fat.
- Foods such as oyako domburi (chicken omelet over rice) and chawan mushi (chicken and shrimp in egg custard) are high in cholesterol, since they contain 1 to 2 eggs per serving.

```
┌─────────────────────────────────────────┐
│        TIPS ON LOWERING SODIUM            │
│ · Japanese food is high in sodium due to  │
│   the soy sauce, MSG (monosodium          │
│   glutamate), and salt used in soups,     │
│   sauces, marinades, cooking broths,      │
│   dipping sauces, and salad dressings.    │
│ · To reduce your sodium intake, order     │
│   grilled seafood, chicken, or steaks     │
│   prepared without marinades, sauces, or  │
│   added salt.                             │
│ · Request plain steamed rice. Use dipping │
│   sauces sparingly, if at all.            │
│ · Sashimi is a low-sodium choice; however,│
│   caution is advised in eating raw fish.  │
└─────────────────────────────────────────┘
```

The following table gives you an idea of the calories, fat, saturated fat, and cholesterol content of selected foods from Japanese cuisine. Whenever possible, several recipes were averaged to obtain the values listed; however, these figures are only estimates, and the content of an actual dish may vary, depending on how the chef prepares it. Within each section—appetizers, sushi and sashimi, entrées, noodles and rice, and sauces—foods are arranged from low to high fat. Usually foods lower in fat are also lower in calories and saturated fat. If you do not see some of the lower-fat foods listed below on a restaurant menu, you may wish to request them.

	Cal	Fat g	Sat g	Chol mg
APPETIZERS				
Sumashi Wan				
Clear soup w/tofu & shrimp	58	2	0	23
Chawan Mushi				
Chicken & shrimp in egg custard	111	5	2	226
Yakitori				
Broiled chicken, scallions &				
chicken livers	275	6	2	319
Agedashi				
Fried tofu in sauce	342	23	3	4

	Cal	Fat g	Sat g	Chol mg
SUSHI AND SASHIMI				
Sliced raw tuna (3 oz)	131	4	1	34
Nigiri Sushi (4 pieces) Vinegared rice & raw fish	186	4	1	40
Makizushi Vinegared rice, omelet & vegetables rolled in seaweed	366	4	1	72
ENTRÉES				
Yosenabe Seafood & vegetables in broth	149	2	0	48
Gyuniku Teriyaki Broiled beef w/teriyaki glaze	323	7	2	113
Shabu Shabu Beef & vegetables cooked in broth	391	14	3	75
Sukiyaki Beef & vegetables cooked in sauce	487	14	3	81
Tonkatsu Breaded pork cutlet	485	30	7	189
Tempura Deep-fried shrimp & vegetables	637	42	10	201
MENRUI (NOODLES) AND **GOHAN (RICE)**				
Su Udon Hot noodles & broth	312	1	0	0
Oyako Domburi Chicken omelet over rice	614	12	4	456
DIPPING SAUCES				
Ponzu for shabu shabu (1 Tbsp)	6	0	0	0
Soy Sauce (1 Tbsp)	10	0	0	0
Tosa Joyu for sashimi (1 Tbsp)	12	0	0	0
Chirizu for yosenabe (1 Tbsp)	14	0	0	0

c = cup; Cal = calories; Chol = cholesterol; diam = diameter; fl oz = fluid ounce; g = gram; lg = large; mayo = mayonnaise; med = medium; mg = milligram; na = not available; oz = ounce; prep = prepared; Sat = saturated fat; sl = slice; sm = small; Tbsp = tablespoon; tr = trace; tsp = teaspoon; w/ = with; w/o = without

MEXICAN CUISINE

Mexican food is gaining in popularity across the United States. Many of the items found on the menu of a Mexican restaurant differ from the dishes you would find in Mexico; these foods are known as TexMex. Some examples of popular TexMex foods are fajitas, nachos, chili con queso, crispy fried tacos, burritos, and chimichangas. Generally TexMex foods contain more cheese and have gravy added to them. In Mexico tamales are usually steamed in the corn husk and served with salsa; the TexMex version is served with gravy.

Entrées served in Mexican restaurants often contain less meat (1 to 2 ounces) than those served in most other types of restaurants. High-fat ingredients, such as cheese, ground meat, and sour cream, are used in many of the dishes. Mexican restaurants differ in the type of fat they use—vegetable oil or lard—to prepare foods such as refried beans and tostadas.

There are two types of Mexican bread—corn tortillas and flour tortillas—used as appetizers, in entrées, and as an accompaniment to the meal. Flour tortillas, which often contain lard, provide more than four times the fat of corn tortillas. Corn tortillas contain no fat unless they are dipped in hot fat for enchiladas or fried, as in tortilla chips or tostadas for chalupas.

MENU TERMS THAT INDICATE HIGH FAT

Carnitas—Fried pieces of beef or pork
Chorizo—Highly seasoned sausage of chopped pork
Quesadilla—Flour or corn tortilla, filled with meat and cheese and fried
Refried beans—Beans mashed and cooked with fat, usually lard

Menu Terms That Indicate High Fat
(*continued*)

Tamale—Dough made with lard or shortening; filled with ground beef, chicken, or pork; wrapped in a corn husk; and steamed

Tostada (or chalupa)—Fried tortilla topped with beans, meat, cheese, lettuce, tomato, sour cream, and/or avocado

TIPS ON ORDERING
LOWER-FAT MEXICAN FOOD

- When you first sit down, request soft or steamed corn tortillas in place of the tortilla chips usually on the table; dip soft corn tortillas in salsa (hot sauce) as an appetizer instead of ordering nachos (fried tortilla chips, topped with cheese, jalapeño peppers, ground beef, and/or refried beans).
- Request that little or no fat be used in cooking fajitas, which are marinated strips of beef or chicken cooked with onion and bell peppers.
- Choose frijoles a la charra or borracho beans rather than refried beans.
- Request that sour cream and cheese be omitted from dishes or served in side dishes so that you can control the amount used.
- Guacamole (puréed avocado with spices), served as a salad or garnish, is low in saturated fat but high in total fat.
- Use salsa, which is fat-free, as a dressing on chicken fajita salad; request a dish of cilantro or jalapeño peppers for extra zest.
- If you order a salad that is served in a fried tortilla shell, think of the shell as a dish and do not eat it.
- Ask if the restaurant has "off the menu" items, such as grilled fish or chicken breast (usually seasoned with onion, cilantro, and Mexican spices).

TIPS ON LOWERING SODIUM

- Request that cheese not be added to food.
- Request soft or steamed corn tortillas to eat with salsa as an appetizer.
- Order grilled chicken, grilled fish, or fajitas, and ask that salt not be used in preparation; you cannot reduce the sodium in foods already prepared, such as enchiladas, burritos, and tacos.
- Select a fajita salad, and use salsa for the dressing instead of chile con queso or salad dressing.

The following table gives you an idea of the calories, fat, saturated fat, and cholesterol content of selected foods from Mexican cuisine. Whenever possible, several recipes were averaged to obtain the values listed; however, these figures are only estimates, and the content of an actual dish may vary, depending on how the chef prepares it. Within each section—appetizers, entrées, accompaniments, and desserts—foods are arranged from low to high fat. Usually foods lower in fat are also lower in calories and saturated fat. If you do not see some of the lower-fat foods listed below on a restaurant menu, you may wish to request them.

	Cal	Fat g	Sat g	Chol mg
APPETIZERS				
Corn tortilla, soft, 5½"	48	1	0	0
Flour tortilla, 8"	126	3	1	3
Ceviche				
Raw fish marinated in lime juice & spices	149	5	1	45
Tortilla Chips (24)	199	9	1	0
Guacamole (½ c)				
Mashed avocado w/onion & spices	164	13	2	0

	Cal	Fat g	Sat g	Chol mg
Fried Nachos (3)				
Tortilla w/meat, refried beans, guacamole, cheese, lettuce & tomato				
w/chicken	246	16	8	42
w/fajita beef	267	19	9	45
w/ground beef	316	23	11	59
Chile con Queso (3 oz)				
Creamy cheese sauce seasoned w/salsa	206	17	10	51
Queso Flameado (7 oz)				
Melted cheese w/sausage	358	30	17	87

ENTRÉES

	Cal	Fat g	Sat g	Chol mg
Chicken Fajita (8 oz)				
Marinated chicken breast w/onions, grilled or broiled	311	6	2	124
Cooked w/fat	362	12	4	124
Taco or Fajita Salad				
Fried tortilla in shape of bowl filled w/tossed salad, meat & accompaniments				
w/grilled chicken only, bowl not eaten	286	11	2	87
w/grilled beef only, bowl not eaten	426	28	9	76
w/grilled chicken, tortilla bowl, guacamole, cheese & sour cream	940	55	21	155
w/grilled beef, tortilla bowl, guacamole, cheese & sour cream	1083	73	28	144

c = cup; Cal = calories; Chol = cholesterol; diam = diameter; fl oz = fluid ounce; g = gram; lg = large; mayo = mayonnaise; med = medium; mg = milligram; na = not available; oz = ounce; prep = prepared; Sat = saturated fat; sl = slice; sm = small; Tbsp = tablespoon; tr = trace; tsp = teaspoon; w/ = with; w/o = without

	Cal	Fat g	Sat g	Chol mg
Entrées *(continued)*				
Enchiladas				
Tortillas dipped in hot oil & wrapped around meat w/gravy on top				
w/chicken (1)	279	16	8	65
w/beef (1)	305	21	9	60
w/ground beef & cheese sauce (1)	320	23	11	67
w/shredded pork (1)	342	24	11	64
w/cheese (2)	379	27	14	59
Tamales, beef (2)	284	19	7	26
Burrito (1)				
Flour tortilla wrapped around assorted fillings, topped w/chili, lettuce, tomato, sour cream & guacamole				
w/refried beans & chili con queso	500	22	10	43
w/chicken & refried beans	603	25	11	90
w/beef, refried beans & chili con queso	630	31	14	81
Beef Fajita (8 oz)				
Marinated skirt steak w/onions, grilled or broiled	507	32	13	127
Cooked w/fat	558	38	14	127
Flauta (1)				
Corn tortilla filled w/meat, rolled up & fried				
w/chicken	490	26	8	76
w/shredded pork	431	28	11	60
w/shredded or ground beef	447	30	12	61
Chimichanga (fried burrito) (1)				
Flour tortilla filled w/meat, rolled up & fried crisp	430	27	8	62
Tacos (beef) (2)				
Fried tortillas folded in half & filled w/meat, lettuce, tomato & cheese	487	32	14	95

	Cal	Fat g	Sat g	Chol mg
Chalupa (1)				
Fried corn tortilla layered w/assorted toppings, cheese, guacamole, lettuce & tomato				
w/chicken	658	40	18	112
w/ground beef	654	43	18	98
w/shredded pork	668	45	19	94
w/sliced beef	746	51	23	118

ACCOMPANIMENTS

	Cal	Fat g	Sat g	Chol mg
Pico de Gallo (½ c)				
Relish of chopped tomatoes, onions, chili peppers, cilantro, lime juice & oil	59	4	1	0
Spanish Rice (1 c)				
Rice fried in oil, then cooked w/spices & tomato	233	4	1	0
Frijoles a la Charra or Borracho Beans (1 c)				
Pinto beans cooked w/bacon	172	6	2	3
Refried Beans (1 c)				
Mashed beans fried in fat, usually lard	515	27	10	24

DESSERTS

	Cal	Fat g	Sat g	Chol mg
Sopapilla (1)				
Dough dropped in hot oil until puffed & golden brown	114	9	2	0
Flan (1)				
Custard w/eggs, milk & sugar, topped w/caramel sauce	362	12	5	305

c = cup; Cal = calories; Chol = cholesterol; diam = diameter; fl oz = fluid ounce; g = gram; lg = large; mayo = mayonnaise; med = medium; mg = milligram; na = not available; oz = ounce; prep = prepared; Sat = saturated fat; sl = slice; sm = small; Tbsp = tablespoon; tr = trace; tsp = teaspoon; w/ = with; w/o = without

THAI CUISINE

Thai food offers an interesting combination of sharply defined flavors: sweet, hot, sour, salty, and bitter. These flavors are blended in some dishes, while in others one flavor predominates. Entrées, especially curries, are often very hot. Rice is served with most Thai meals to offset the spicy-hot chilies. Most Thai recipes contain sugar, and many incorporate fish sauce, made by fermenting fish with salt. Thai salads, which often combine raw vegetables with shrimp, squid, or beef, are very popular.

MENU TERMS THAT INDICATE HIGH FAT

Coconut milk or coconut cream—Used to prepare curry, sauces, custards, and other desserts

Peanut sauce—Sauce of coconut milk, fish sauce, sugar, and peanuts, eaten with most dishes

---

TIPS ON ORDERING LOWER-FAT THAI FOOD

- Order fresh spring rolls rather than fried spring rolls.
- Select stir-fried entrées instead of curry.
- Eat steamed rice rather than fried rice.
- Choose dishes without peanuts and cashews, which are high in fat.

TIPS ON LOWERING SODIUM

- Choose cooked-to-order dishes, and ask that MSG and salt be omitted during food preparation.
- Eat steamed rice, which is salt-free, instead of fried rice.
- Add very little or no high-sodium fish sauce and soy sauce to food.

The following table gives you an idea of the calories, fat, saturated fat, and cholesterol content of selected foods from Thai cuisine. Whenever possible, several recipes were averaged to obtain the values listed; however, these figures are only estimates, and the content of an actual dish may vary, depending on how the chef prepares it. Within each section—appetizers, salads, entrées, accompaniments, sauces and condiments, and desserts—foods are arranged from low to high fat. Usually foods lower in fat are also lower in calories and saturated fat. If you do not see some of the lower-fat foods listed below on a restaurant menu, you may wish to request them.

	Cal	Fat g	Sat g	Chol mg
APPETIZERS				
Gaeng Liang				
Vegetable soup w/shrimp	92	1	0	108
Tom Yam Goong				
Hot & sour shrimp soup	83	1	0	82
Goong Kratiem Prik Thai				
Marinated & sautéed shrimp	80	2	0	107
Poh Taek				
Seafood combination soup	186	3	1	154
Nuea Satay				
Beef cooked on skewer	98	5	2	32
Mee Grob				
Crispy noodles w/fried egg	234	10	2	107
Gaeng Jued Woon Sen				
Glass noodle soup	209	11	4	35
Khao Tom Moo				
Rice soup w/pork	224	11	4	35
Po Pia Sod (3)				
Fresh spring rolls w/sausage, tofu & spinach (not fried)	251	15	5	33

c = cup; Cal = calories; Chol = cholesterol; diam = diameter; fl oz = fluid ounce; g = gram; lg = large; mayo = mayonnaise; med = medium; mg = milligram; na = not available; oz = ounce; prep = prepared; Sat = saturated fat; sl = slice; sm = small; Tbsp = tablespoon; tr = trace; tsp = teaspoon; w/ = with; w/o = without

	Cal	Fat g	Sat g	Chol mg
Appetizers *(continued)*				
Tom Kha Gai				
Chicken coconut soup	324	25	20	40
Po Pia Taud (5)				
Spring rolls w/pork, vegetables & egg (fried)	435	29	7	142

SALADS

	Cal	Fat g	Sat g	Chol mg
Yam Po Taek				
Seafood salad	151	2	1	135
Yam Nuea				
Beef salad	197	5	2	75
Laab Nuea				
Ground beef salad	267	16	6	56

ENTRÉES

	Cal	Fat g	Sat g	Chol mg
Kanaa Namman Hoi				
Stir-fried broccoli w/oyster sauce	126	7	1	0
Nuea Pad Kanaa				
Sautéed beef w/broccoli	174	9	2	38
Nuea Pad Prik				
Pepper steak	295	15	3	75
Gai Ob Surat				
Thai baked chicken	328	17	5	125
Gai Yang				
Barbecued chicken	328	17	5	125
Pad Thai				
Stir-fried Thai noodles	405	18	3	84
Pad Pak Tow-Hoo				
Fried tofu stir-fried w/vegetables	268	19	3	0
Gai Pad Med Ma-Muang Himapan				
Cashew chicken	410	27	5	68
Gaeng Ped Gai				
Red curry chicken	427	29	24	62
Gaeng Keow Wan Gai				
Green curry w/chicken & Thai eggplant	602	37	30	64

	Cal	Fat g	Sat g	Chol mg
ACCOMPANIMENTS				
Steamed White Rice (1 c)	241	0	0	0
Khao Pad Moo Fried rice w/pork	550	18	5	157
Thai Fried Rice w/Bacon	418	21	4	168
Khao Ob Sapparod Rice w/pineapple, chicken & coconut milk	898	48	27	34
SAUCES AND CONDIMENTS				
Black Chili Paste (1 Tbsp) Blended dip w/fried chili peppers	21	1	0	15
Peanut Sauce (1 Tbsp) Ground peanuts w/coconut milk, red curry paste & fish sauce	45	4	2	0
Chopped Peanuts (1 Tbsp)	48	4	1	0
DESSERTS				
Khao Newo Kaew Sweet sticky rice	428	12	10	0
Sangkaya Thai custard w/egg & coconut cream	459	22	15	319
Ta-Go Rice pudding w/coconut cream topping	671	30	27	0
Khao Neow Ma-Muang Sweet rice w/mango	941	31	27	0
Gluay Kaeg Banana slices dipped in coconut batter & fried	659	39	12	0

c = cup; Cal = calories; Chol = cholesterol; diam = diameter; fl oz = fluid ounce; g = gram; lg = large; mayo = mayonnaise; med = medium; mg = milligram; na = not available; oz = ounce; prep = prepared; Sat = saturated fat; sl = slice; sm = small; Tbsp = tablespoon; tr = trace; tsp = teaspoon; w/ = with; w/o = without

VIETNAMESE CUISINE

Vietnamese cuisine reflects the influence of the French, who ruled Vietnam for more than a century; many dishes are similar to Chinese and Thai food, but tend to have less intense, more subtle flavors. Contrasting textures, such as combining fresh greens and/or crunchy peanuts with cooked food, are characteristic of many Vietnamese dishes. Vietnamese food tends to be low in fat, and small amounts of vegetable oil rather than lard are used for stir-frying. All of the regional Vietnamese cuisines include fish, shellfish, fresh vegetables, and barbecued dishes.

Nuoc mam is one of the most characteristic ingredients of Vietnamese cuisine. It is commercially prepared by layering fresh anchovies with salt, allowing them to ferment, and draining off the sauce. When lime juice, chilies, sugar, garlic, and vinegar are added to nuoc mam, it is called nuoc cham. Nuoc mam, which is very high in sodium, is used in place of salt at the table and in cooking.

MENU TERMS THAT INDICATE HIGH FAT

Curry—Sauce made with coconut milk or heavy cream

Peanut Sauce—Sauce of crushed peanuts, peanut oil, broth, tomato paste, and chili peppers, served with most appetizers and entrées

---

TIPS ON ORDERING LOWER-FAT VIETNAMESE FOOD

· Eat steamed rice rather than fried rice with your entrée.
· When dining with a group, order one fewer entrée than the number of people and share.

The following table gives you an idea of the calories, fat, saturated fat, and cholesterol content of selected foods from Vietnamese cuisine. Whenever possible, several recipes were averaged to obtain the values listed; however, these figures are only estimates, and the content of an actual dish may vary, depending on how the chef prepares it. Within each section—appetizers, entrées, sauces and accompaniments, and desserts—foods are arranged from low to high fat. Usually foods lower in fat are also lower in calories and saturated fat. If you do not see some of the lower-fat foods listed below on a restaurant menu, you may wish to request them.

	Cal	Fat g	Sat g	Chol mg

APPETIZERS

	Cal	Fat g	Sat g	Chol mg
Canh Chua Tom Spicy & sour shrimp soup	118	6	1	54

Goi Cuon (2)
   Fresh spring roll: cold shrimp,
   pork & vegetables rolled in
   rice paper
	306	14	4	96

Cha Gio (6 sm rolls) Fried spring roll	480	30	6	102

Banh Michien Voitom (4 pieces)
   Shrimp toast: bread topped
   w/shrimp paste & fried
	450	40	6	30

ENTRÉES

	Cal	Fat g	Sat g	Chol mg
Ca Hap Steamed whole fish	225	3	1	131

Ech Kho Xa Ot
   Frog legs simmered w/lemon
   grass & chili pepper
	197	4	1	56

Ca Kho To
   Fish simmered w/caramel sauce
   in clay pot
	486	5	1	216

Bo Xa Lui Nuong
   Grilled beef w/lemon grass
   wrapped in rice paper
   w/vegetables
	363	9	2	73

Cua Rang Muoi Fried crab w/salt & pepper	174	12	2	78
Muc Xao Cai Chua Stir-fried squid w/vegetables	303	16	3	271

Bo Nhung Giam
   Beef fondue in broth, wrapped
   in rice paper w/vegetables &
   peanuts
	397	19	4	75

Bun Cha
   Grilled pork & beef patties
   served w/vegetables & rice
   vermicelli
	604	26	10	93

Nem Nuong
   Grilled meatballs w/fresh
   vegetables wrapped in rice
   paper
	644	27	9	126

	Cal	Fat g	Sat g	Chol mg
Heo Xao Chua Ngot				
Sweet-and-sour pork	519	29	6	71
Boluc Lac				
Sautéed spicy beef salad served warm over lettuce w/vinaigrette dressing	458	32	5	75
Vit Quay				
Roast duck, BBQ style	662	33	8	120
Ca-Ri Ga				
Chicken curry	830	53	31	98

SAUCES AND ACCOMPANIMENTS

	Cal	Fat g	Sat g	Chol mg
Nuoc Mam				
Fish sauce (1 Tbsp)	7	0	0	0
Bean sprouts (1 c)	11	0	0	0
Mam Nem (1 Tbsp)				
Anchovy & pineapple sauce	14	0	0	0
Steamed White Rice (1 c)	241	0	0	0
Peanut Sauce (1 Tbsp)				
Peanuts, oil & spices	34	2	0	0
Peanuts, chopped (1 Tbsp)	48	4	1	0

DESSERTS

	Cal	Fat g	Sat g	Chol mg
Lychee (½ c)				
Fruit in syrup	57	0	0	0
Che Hot Sen That Tranh				
Iced jelly, lotus seeds & mung beans in coconut syrup	532	13	11	0
Banh Dua Ca Ra Men				
Coconut flan w/caramel	292	18	13	177

BEVERAGES

	Cal	Fat g	Sat g	Chol mg
Ca Phe Sua Da				
French coffee w/condensed milk over ice	91	3	2	10

c = cup; Cal = calories; Chol = cholesterol; diam = diameter; fl oz = fluid ounce; g = gram; lg = large; mayo = mayonnaise; med = medium; mg = milligram; na = not available; oz = ounce; prep = prepared; Sat = saturated fat; sl = slice; sm = small; Tbsp = tablespoon; tr = trace; tsp = teaspoon; w/ = with; w/o = without

Chapter 4

Fast Food

With the fast-paced lifestyle of many Americans, food that can be obtained quickly and easily has become very popular. Although much of the fast food presently available is high in calories, fat, saturated fat, and sodium, some selections are lower. Within each section—breakfast items, salads, hamburgers, sandwiches, other entrées, side orders, and desserts—foods are listed from low to high fat. Those foods providing less fat are the preferred choices. The fast food beverage category contains values only for milkshakes. Soft drinks, juice, milk, coffee, and tea are basically the same anyplace they are sold, with only the serving size varying (see Beverages, page 41). Salad dressings are shown on page 20 instead of with the information for each fast food chain, so be sure to add in the values for any dressing you put on your salad.

The tips on lowering fat provided throughout this book also apply to fast food. See page 32 for pizza and page 26 for sandwiches (including burgers).

**TIPS ON ORDERING
LOWER-FAT FAST FOOD**

- **Order a regular or small hamburger without cheese instead of a larger hamburger or quarter-pounder.**
- **Sliced meat (roast beef or turkey) and grilled chicken sandwiches are usually lower in fat than sandwiches containing ground meat (hamburger and meatball subs), luncheon meat (bologna and salami subs), and/or cheese (grilled cheese, cheeseburger, and meat and cheese subs).**

Tips on Ordering Lower-Fat Fast Food
(*continued*)

- Choose a salad (without cheese, croutons, or bacon) with lite dressing instead of French fries.
- Request pretzels instead of chips.
- Request juice, low-fat milk, or cola (regular or diet) rather than a milkshake.

TIP ON LOWERING SODIUM

- Request lettuce, tomato, and onions on sandwiches instead of condiments that, although low in fat, are high in sodium; these include catsup, mustard, pickles, and steak sauce.

ARBY'S INC.

	Cal	Fat g	Sat g	Chol mg
BREAKFAST ITEMS				
Blueberry Muffin	240	7	1	22
Cinnamon Nut Danish	360	11	1	0
Biscuit, plain	280	15	3	0
w/ham	323	17	4	21
w/bacon	318	18	4	8
w/sausage	460	32	9	60
Croissant, plain	260	16	10	49
w/ham & cheese	345	21	12	90
w/bacon & egg	430	30	15	245
w/mushroom & cheese	493	38	15	116
w/sausage & egg	519	39	19	271
Egg Platter w/Potato Cake & Blueberry Muffin	460	24	7	346
w/ham	518	26	8	374
w/bacon	593	33	9	458
w/sausage	640	41	13	406
Toastix (1 ord)	420	25	5	20
SOUPS (8 oz)				
Old Fashioned Chicken Noodle	99	2	1	25
Lumberjack Mixed Vegetable	89	4	2	4
Cream of Broccoli	166	7	4	24
Potato with Bacon	184	9	4	20
Boston Clam Chowder	193	10	5	26
Wisconsin Cheese	281	18	9	32
SALADS				
Side	25	0	0	0
Garden	117	5	3	12
Roast Chicken	204	7	3	43
Chef	205	10	4	126
SANDWICHES				
Light Menu Sandwich				
Roast Turkey Deluxe	260	6	2	33
Roast Chicken Deluxe	276	7	2	33
Roast Beef Deluxe	294	10	4	42

	Cal	Fat g	Sat g	Chol mg
Roast Beef				
Junior	233	11	4	22
French Dip	368	15	6	43
Arby Q	389	15	6	29
Reg	383	18	7	43
French Dip 'N Swiss	429	19	9	67
Philly Beef 'N Swiss	467	25	10	53
Giant	544	26	11	72
Beef 'N Cheddar	508	27	8	52
Super	552	28	8	43
Bac 'N Cheddar Deluxe	512	32	9	38
Chicken				
Grilled Barbeque	386	13	4	43
Grilled Deluxe	430	20	4	44
Breast Fillet	445	23	3	45
Roast Chicken Club	503	27	7	46
Cordon Bleu	518	27	5	92
Ham 'N Cheese	355	14	5	55
Sub Shop				
Turkey	486	19	5	51
Roast Beef	623	32	12	73
Tuna	663	37	8	43
Italian	671	39	13	69
Fish Fillet	526	27	7	44

SIDE ORDERS

	Cal	Fat g	Sat g	Chol mg
Baked Potato, plain	240	2	0	0
Broccoli 'N Cheddar	417	18	7	22
w/Butter or Margarine & Sour Cream	463	25	12	40
Mushroom 'N Cheese	515	27	6	47
Deluxe	621	36	18	58
Potato Cakes (1 ord)	204	12	2	0
French Fries (1 ord)	246	13	3	0
Curly	337	18	7	0
Cheddar	399	22	9	9

c = cup; Cal = calories; Chol = cholesterol; diam = diameter; fl oz = fluid ounce; g = gram; lg = large; mayo = mayonnaise; med = medium; mg = milligram; na = not available; ord = order; oz = ounce; pkt = packet; reg = regular; Sat = saturated fat; sl = slice; sm = small; Tbsp = tablespoon; tr = trace; tsp = teaspoon; w/ = with; w/o = without

	Cal	Fat g	Sat g	Chol mg
SAUCES AND CONDIMENTS				
Au Jus (4 oz)	7	0	0	0
Arby's Sauce (½ oz)	15	0	0	0
Horsey Sauce (½ oz)	55	5	2	1
DESSERTS				
Chocolate Chip Cookie (1)	130	4	2	0
Turnover				
Cherry	280	18	5	0
Apple	303	18	7	0
Blueberry	320	19	6	0
Polar Swirl				
Butterfinger	457	18	8	28
Snickers	511	19	7	33
Oreo	482	20	10	35
Heath	543	22	5	39
Peanut Butter Cup	517	24	8	34
Cheese Cake (1 ord)	306	23	7	95
BEVERAGES				
Shake				
Jamoca	368	11	3	35
Vanilla	330	12	4	32
Chocolate	451	12	3	36

BASKIN-ROBBINS

	Cal	Fat g	Sat g	Chol mg
FROZEN DAIRY DESSERTS				
Fat Free Frozen Dairy Dessert (1 Jr. scoop = 2½ oz)				
Caramel Banana	100	0	0	1
Chocolate Vanilla	100	0	0	0
Jamoca Swirl & Just Peachy	100	0	0	2
Pineapple Cheesecake	110	0	0	0
Chocolate Wonder	120	0	0	1
Sugar Free Frozen Dairy Dessert (1 Jr. scoop)				
Chunky Banana & Strawberry	80	1	1	3
Pineapple Coconut	90	1	1	3
Cherry Cordial	100	1	1	3
Thin Mint Chip & Jamoca Swiss Almond	90	2	1	4
Chocolate Chip	100	2	1	4
Light Frozen Dairy Dessert (1 Jr. scoop)				
Strawberry Royale	110	3	2	9
Vanilla Fudge	110	4	3	11
Double Raspberry	120	4	3	9
Espresso 'N Cream	120	5	3	12
Chocolate Caramel Nut	130	5	3	8
Almond Buttercrunch	130	6	4	12
Praline Dream	130	6	4	11
FROZEN NOVELTIES				
Sundae Bar				
Light Chocolate w/Caramel Ribbon	150	5	na	11
Strawberry Royal	280	9	na	21
Jamoca Almond Fudge	300	13	na	24
Pralines 'N Cream	310	13	na	30
Chillyburger				
Very Berry Strawberry	230	9	na	23
Vanilla	240	11	na	29
Mint Chocolate Chip	260	12	na	26
Chocolate Chip	270	12	na	26

c = cup; Cal = calories; Chol = cholesterol; diam = diameter; fl oz = fluid ounce; g = gram; lg = large; mayo = mayonnaise; med = medium; mg = milligram; na = not available; ord = order; oz = ounce; pkt = packet; reg = regular; Sat = saturated fat; sl = slice; sm = small; Tbsp = tablespoon; tr = trace; tsp = teaspoon; w/ = with; w/o = without

	Cal	Fat g	Sat g	Chol mg
Frozen Novelties *(continued)*				
Tiny Toon Adventures Ice Cream Bar				
Strawberry	210	13	na	15
Vanilla	210	14	na	18
Chocolate Chip & Mint Chocolate Chip	230	15	na	17

FROZEN YOGURT

	Cal	Fat g	Sat g	Chol mg
Truly Free (½ c)				
Cafe Mocha & Wild Cherry	70	0	0	0
Non-Fat (1 Jr. scoop)				
Chocolate, Strawberry & Vanilla	110	0	0	0
Lowfat (1 reg scoop = 4 oz)				
Raspberry	120	2	na	5
Vanilla	120	2	na	6
Chocolate	140	2	na	6

ICE CREAM

	Cal	Fat g	Sat g	Chol mg
Deluxe Ice Cream (1 reg scoop)				
Very Berry Strawberry	220	10	6	30
Cherries Jubilee	240	11	na	35
Jamoca	240	13	8	41
Vanilla	240	14	9	52
Tiny Toon Crunch	250	14	9	43
Chocolate	270	14	9	37
Jamoca Almond Fudge	270	14	9	32
Pralines 'N Cream & World Class Chocolate	280	14	9	36
Rocky Road	300	14	9	32
Chocolate Chip & Mint Chocolate Chip	260	15	10	40
Chocolate Fudge	290	15	10	41
German Chocolate Cake	310	15	10	32
Chocolate Mousse	320	16	11	32
Cookies 'N Cream	280	17	11	39
Butter Pecan	280	18	12	40
French Vanilla	280	18	12	90
Pistachio-Almond	290	18	12	39
Chocolate Almond	300	18	12	34
Fudge Brownie	320	18	12	36
Peanut Butter 'N Chocolate	330	20	13	33

	Cal	Fat g	Sat g	Chol mg
International Creams (1 reg scoop)				
Kahlua 'N Cream	270	14	10	15
Chocolate Raspberry Truffle	310	17	11	45

ICE CREAM CONES

Sugar Cone	60	1	na	0
Waffle Cone	140	2	na	0

ICES AND SHERBETS

Soft Serve Sorbet, Strawberry (½ c)	100	0	0	0
Daiquiri Ice (1 reg scoop)	140	0	0	0
Sherbet, Orange & Rainbow (1 reg scoop)	160	2	na	6

c = cup; Cal = calories; Chol = cholesterol; diam = diameter; fl oz = fluid ounce; g = gram; lg = large; mayo = mayonnaise; med = medium; mg = milligram; na = not available; ord = order; oz = ounce; pkt = packet; reg = regular; Sat = saturated fat; sl = slice; sm = small; Tbsp = tablespoon; tr = trace; tsp = teaspoon; w/ = with; w/o = without

BURGER KING

	Cal	Fat g	Sat g	Chol mg
BREAKFAST ITEMS				
Breakfast Taco w/Egg & Cheese	232	na	na	na
w/Potato	249	na	na	na
w/Sausage	273	na	na	na
Bagel	272	6	1	29
w/Cream Cheese	370	16	6	58
Croissant	180	10	2	4
Hash Browns (1 ord)	213	12	3	0
Mini Muffins (1 ord)				
Raisin Oat Bran	291	12	2	0
Blueberry	292	14	3	72
Lemon Poppyseed	318	18	3	72
Danish				
Apple Cinnamon	390	13	3	19
Cheese	406	16	5	7
Cinnamon Raisin	449	18	4	15
Bagel Sandwich w/Egg & Cheese	407	16	5	247
w/Ham	438	17	6	266
w/Bacon	453	20	7	252
w/Sausage	626	36	12	293
Biscuit	332	17	3	2
w/Bacon	378	20	5	8
w/Bacon & Egg	467	27	7	213
w/Sausage	478	29	8	33
w/Sausage & Egg	568	36	10	238
Croissan'wich w/Egg & Cheese	315	20	7	222
w/Ham	346	22	7	236
w/Bacon	353	23	8	230
w/Sausage	534	40	14	258
French Toast Sticks (1 ord)	440	27	7	0
Scrambled Egg Platter	549	34	9	365
w/Bacon	610	39	11	373
w/Sausage	768	53	15	412
SALADS				
Side	25	0	0	0
Chunky Chicken	142	4	1	49

	Cal	Fat g	Sat g	Chol mg
Garden	95	5	3	15
Chef	178	9	4	103

HAMBURGERS

	Cal	Fat g	Sat g	Chol mg
Hamburger	260	10	4	30
Deluxe	344	19	6	43
Cheeseburger	300	14	6	45
Deluxe	390	23	8	56
Burger Buddies (1 ord)	349	17	7	52
Double Cheeseburger	450	25	12	90
Mushroom Swiss	473	27	12	95
Bacon	470	28	13	100
Barbecue Bacon	536	31	14	105
Bacon Deluxe	530	33	14	100
Whopper	570	31	10	80
w/Cheese	660	38	15	105
Double Whopper	800	48	18	160
w/Cheese	890	55	22	185

SANDWICHES

	Cal	Fat g	Sat g	Chol mg
BK Broiler Chicken	280	10	2	50
Ocean Catch Fish Filet	450	28	7	30
Chicken	620	32	7	45

SIDE ORDERS

	Cal	Fat g	Sat g	Chol mg
Chicken Tenders (1 ord = 6 pieces)	236	13	3	38
Apple Pie (1)	320	14	4	0
Onion Rings (1 ord)	339	19	5	0
French Fries (1 med)	372	20	5	0

c = cup; Cal = calories; Chol = cholesterol; diam = diameter; fl oz = fluid ounce; g = gram; lg = large; mayo = mayonnaise; med = medium; mg = milligram; na = not available; ord = order; oz = ounce; pkt = packet; reg = regular; Sat = saturated fat; sl = slice; sm = small; Tbsp = tablespoon; tr = trace; tsp = teaspoon; w/ = with; w/o = without

	Cal	Fat g	Sat g	Chol mg
SAUCES AND CONDIMENTS				
Bull's Eye Barbecue Sauce (½ oz)	22	0	0	0
Dipping Sauce (1 oz = 2 Tbsp)				
Barbecue	36	0	0	0
Sweet & Sour	45	0	0	0
A.M. Express	84	0	0	0
Honey	91	0	0	0
Ranch	171	18	3	0
BK Broiler Sauce (1 pkt)	37	4	1	5
BEVERAGES				
Shake (1 med)				
Chocolate	326	10	6	31
Vanilla	334	10	6	33
Strawberry w/syrup	394	10	6	33
Chocolate w/syrup	409	11	6	33

CAPTAIN D'S

	Cal	Fat g	Sat g	Chol mg
ENTRÉES				
Chicken Dinner w/Rice, Green Beans, Breadstick & Salad	414	8	na	71
Shrimp Dinner w/Rice, Green Beans, Breadstick & Salad	457	9	na	191
Orange Roughy Dinner w/Rice Green Beans, Breadstick & Salad	537	19	na	39
Baked Fish Dinner w/Rice, Green Beans, Breadstick & Salad	659	30	na	54
SIDE ORDERS				
Rice (1 ord)	124	0	0	0
Dinner Salad (1 ord)	27	1	0	1
White Beans (1 ord)	126	1	0	2
Green Beans, Seasoned (1 ord)	46	2	na	4
Breadsticks (6)	545	7	na	0
French Fried Potatoes (1 ord)	302	10	na	0
Cole Slaw (1 ord)	158	12	na	16
Fried Okra (1 ord)	300	16	na	0
Cracklins (1 oz)	218	17	na	0
Hushpuppies (6)	756	25	na	0
SAUCES (1 oz)				
Sweet & Sour Sauce	52	0	na	0
Cocktail Sauce	34	<1	0	0
Tartar Sauce	75	7	na	10
DESSERTS (1 ord)				
Chocolate Cake	303	10	na	20
Lemon Pie	351	10	na	45
Pecan Pie	458	20	na	4
Carrot Cake	434	23	na	32
Cheesecake	420	31	na	141

c = cup; Cal = calories; Chol = cholesterol; diam = diameter; fl oz = fluid ounce; g = gram; lg = large; mayo = mayonnaise; med = medium; mg = milligram; na = not available; ord = order; oz = ounce; pkt = packet; reg = regular; Sat = saturated fat; sl = slice; sm = small; Tbsp = tablespoon; tr = trace; tsp = teaspoon; w/ = with; w/o = without

CARL'S JR.

	Cal	Fat g	Sat g	Chol mg
BREAKFAST ITEMS				
Bacon (2 strips)	45	4	1	5
English Muffin w/Margarine	190	5	1	0
Muffin				
Bran	310	7	0	60
Blueberry	340	9	1	45
Scrambled Eggs (1 ord)	120	9	4	245
Sunrise Sandwich	300	13	6	160
Hash Brown Nuggets (1 ord)	270	17	4	5
Sausage (1 patty)	190	18	5	30
Cinnamon Roll	460	18	1	0
French Toast Dips, syrup not included (1 ord)	450	20	6	4
Hot Cakes w/Margarine, syrup not included (1 ord)	510	24	5	10
Breakfast Burrito	430	26	12	285
SALADS				
Salad-To-Go				
Garden	50	3	2	5
Chicken	200	8	4	70
ENTRÉES				
"Great Stuff" Potato				
Lite Potato	290	1	0	0
Sour Cream & Chive	470	19	7	20
Chili	500	26	11	50
Broccoli & Cheese	590	31	11	25
Cheese	690	36	15	40
Bacon & Cheese	730	43	15	45
Chicken Strips (6)	260	19	5	25
HAMBURGERS				
Hamburger	320	14	5	35
Carl's Original	460	20	9	50
Famous Star	610	38	13	50
Super Star	820	53	24	105
Western Bacon Cheeseburger	730	39	20	90
Double	1030	63	32	145

	Cal	Fat g	Sat g	Chol mg
SANDWICHES				
Charbroiled BBQ Chicken	310	6	2	30
Club				
Turkey	530	23	6	60
Charbroiled Chicken	570	29	8	60
Roast Beef	620	34	11	45
Santa Fe Chicken	530	29	7	85
Carl's Catch Fish	560	30	4	5
SIDE ORDERS				
French Fries (reg size)	420	20	5	0
CrissCut	330	22	3	tr
Fried Zucchini (1 ord)	390	23	6	0
Onion Rings (1 ord)	520	26	6	0
SAUCES AND CONDIMENTS				
Salsa	8	0	0	0
DESSERTS				
Chocolate Cake	300	11	3	25
Cheesecake	310	17	8	60
Chocolate Chip Cookie (1)	330	17	7	5
Fudge Moussecake	400	23	11	110
BEVERAGES				
Shake (reg)	350	7	4	15

c = cup; Cal = calories; Chol = cholesterol; diam = diameter; fl oz = fluid ounce; g = gram; lg = large; mayo = mayonnaise; med = medium; mg = milligram; na = not available; ord = order; oz = ounce; pkt = packet; reg = regular; Sat = saturated fat; sl = slice; sm = small; Tbsp = tablespoon; tr = trace; tsp = teaspoon; w/ = with; w/o = without

DAIRY QUEEN

	Cal	Fat g	Sat g	Chol mg
DESSERTS				
Yogurt Cone, reg	180	1	0	5
Lg	260	1	0	5
Cup of Yogurt, reg	170	1	0	5
Lg	230	1	0	5
Sundae				
Strawberry Yogurt, reg	200	1	0	5
Chocolate, reg	300	7	5	20
Strawberry Waffle Cone	350	12	5	20
Chocolate, lg	540	14	8	45
Strawberry Breeze, sm	400	1	0	5
Reg	590	1	0	5
DQ Sandwich	140	4	2	5
Vanilla Cone, sm	140	4	3	15
Reg	230	7	5	20
Lg	340	10	7	30
Chocolate Cone, reg	230	7	5	20
Lg	350	11	8	30
Banana Split	510	11	8	30
Heath Breeze, sm	450	12	3	10
Lg	680	21	6	15
Strawberry Blizzard, sm	500	12	8	35
Reg	740	16	11	50
Dilly Bar	210	13	6	10
Big Scoop				
QC Vanilla	300	14	9	35
QC Chocolate	310	14	10	35
Chocolate Dipped Cone, reg	330	16	8	20
DQ Frozen Cake Slice	380	18	8	20
Nutty Double Fudge	580	22	10	35
Heath Blizzard, sm	560	23	11	40
Reg	820	36	17	60
Buster Bar	450	29	9	15
Hot Fudge Brownie Delight	710	29	14	35
Peanut Buster Parfait	710	32	10	30

	Cal	Fat g	Sat g	Chol mg
BEVERAGES				
Mr. Misty, reg	250	0	0	0
Vanilla Shake, reg	520	14	8	45
Lg	600	16	10	50
Vanilla Malt, reg	610	14	8	45

c = cup; Cal = calories; Chol = cholesterol; diam = diameter; fl oz = fluid ounce; g = gram; lg = large; mayo = mayonnaise; med = medium; mg = milligram; na = not available; ord = order; oz = ounce; pkt = packet; reg = regular; Sat = saturated fat; sl = slice; sm = small; Tbsp = tablespoon; tr = trace; tsp = teaspoon; w/ = with; w/o = without

DOMINO'S

	Cal	Fat g	Sat g	Chol mg
PIZZA				
Vegetable Pizza w/Mushrooms, Onions, Green Peppers & Olives (⅛ of 12″ pizza)	204	5	3	9
Pepperoni Pizza (⅛ of 12″ pizza)	219	7	4	14

DUNKIN' DONUTS

	Cal	Fat g	Sat g	Chol mg
COOKIES (1)				
Oatmeal Pecan Raisin	200	9	na	25
Chocolate Chunk	200	10	na	30
w/Nuts	210	11	na	30
CROISSANTS (1)				
Plain	310	19	na	0
Almond	420	27	na	0
Chocolate	440	29	na	0
DOUGHNUTS (1)				
Filled				
Blueberry	210	8	na	0
Jelly	220	9	na	0
Bavarian w/Chocolate Frosting	240	11	na	0
Apple w/Cinnamon Sugar	250	11	na	0
Lemon	260	12	na	0
Yeast				
Glazed	200	9	na	0
Chocolate Frosted	200	10	na	0
Glazed				
Buttermilk	290	14	na	10
Whole Wheat	330	18	na	0
Chocolate	324	21	na	0
Plain Cake	270	17	na	0
MUFFINS (1)				
Blueberry	280	8	na	30
Apple N' Spice	300	8	na	25
Cranberry Nut	290	9	na	25
Bran w/Raisins	310	9	na	15
Banana Nut	310	10	na	30
Oat Bran	330	11	na	0
Corn	340	12	na	40
SWEET ROLLS (1)				
French Cruller, Glazed	140	8	na	30
Coffee Roll, Glazed	280	12	na	0

c = cup; Cal = calories; Chol = cholesterol; diam = diameter; fl oz = fluid ounce; g = gram; lg = large; mayo = mayonnaise; med = medium; mg = milligram; na = not available; ord = order; oz = ounce; pkt = packet; reg = regular; Sat = saturated fat; sl = slice; sm = small; Tbsp = tablespoon; tr = trace; tsp = teaspoon; w/ = with; w/o = without

GODFATHER'S

	Cal	Fat g	Sat g	Chol mg
PIZZA				
Original Crust Pizza, Cheese				
¼ Mini	138	4	na	13
⅙ Sm	239	7	na	25
⅛ Med	242	7	na	22
1/10 Lg	271	8	na	28
Original Crust Pizza, Combo				
¼ Mini	164	5	na	17
⅙ Sm	299	11	na	37
⅛ Med	318	12	na	38
1/10 Lg	332	12	na	39
Golden Crust Pizza, Cheese				
⅙ Sm	213	8	na	19
⅛ Med	229	9	na	19
1/10 Lg	261	11	na	23
Golden Crust Pizza, Combo				
⅙ Sm	273	12	na	31
⅛ Med	283	13	na	29
1/10 Lg	322	15	na	34

HARDEE'S

	Cal	Fat g	Sat g	Chol mg
BREAKFAST ITEMS				
Three Pancakes (1 ord)	280	2	1	15
w/2 Bacon Strips	350	9	3	25
w/1 Sausage Pattie	430	16	6	40
Hash Rounds (1 ord)	230	14	3	0
Biscuit (1)				
Ham	320	16	2	15
Cinnamon 'N' Raisin	320	17	5	0
Rise 'N' Shine	320	18	3	0
Country Ham	350	18	3	25
Ham & Egg	370	19	4	160
Bacon	360	21	4	10
Country Ham & Egg	400	22	4	175
Chicken	430	22	4	45
Ham, Egg & Cheese	420	23	6	170
Bacon & Egg	410	24	5	155
'N' Gravy	440	24	6	15
Canadian Rise 'N' Shine	470	27	8	180
Sausage	440	28	7	25
Bacon, Egg & Cheese	460	28	8	165
Steak	500	29	7	30
Sausage & Egg	490	31	8	170
Steak & Egg	550	32	8	175
Big Country Breakfast (1 ord)				
Ham	620	33	7	325
Country Ham	670	38	9	345
Bacon	660	40	10	305
Sausage	850	57	16	340
SALADS				
Side	20	1	0	0
Chicken 'N' Pasta	230	3	1	55
Garden	210	14	8	105
Chef	240	15	9	115

c = cup; Cal = calories; Chol = cholesterol; diam = diameter; fl oz = fluid ounce; g = gram; lg = large; mayo = mayonnaise; med = medium; mg = milligram; na = not available; ord = order; oz = ounce; pkt = packet; reg = regular; Sat = saturated fat; sl = slice; sm = small; Tbsp = tablespoon; tr = trace; tsp = teaspoon; w/ = with; w/o = without

	Cal	Fat g	Sat g	Chol mg
HAMBURGERS				
Hamburger	270	10	4	20
Cheeseburger	320	14	7	30
Mushroom 'N' Swiss	490	27	13	70
Quarter-Pound	500	29	14	70
Bacon	610	39	16	80
Big Burger				
Twin	450	25	11	55
Deluxe	500	30	12	70
SANDWICHES				
Roast Beef, reg	260	9	4	35
Big	300	11	5	45
Grilled Chicken	310	9	1	60
Hot Ham 'N' Cheese	330	12	5	65
Chicken Fillet	370	13	2	55
Turkey Club	390	16	4	70
All Beef Hot Dog	300	17	8	25
Fisherman's Fillet	500	24	6	70
SIDE ORDERS				
French Fries, reg	230	11	2	0
Crispy Curls (1 ord)	300	16	3	0
Lg	360	17	3	0
Big Fry	500	23	5	0
Chicken Stix (1 ord = 9)	310	14	3	55
DESSERTS				
Cool Twist Cone				
Vanilla	190	6	4	15
Vanilla/Chocolate	190	6	4	20
Chocolate	200	6	4	20
Cool Twist Sundae				
Strawberry	260	8	5	15
Caramel	330	10	5	20
Hot Fudge	320	12	6	25
Apple Turnover	270	12	4	0
Big Cookie (1)	250	13	4	5

	Cal	Fat g	Sat g	Chol mg
BEVERAGES				
Shake				
Strawberry	440	8	5	40
Chocolate	460	8	5	45
Vanilla	400	9	6	50

c = cup; Cal = calories; Chol = cholesterol; diam = diameter; fl oz = fluid ounce; g = gram; lg = large; mayo = mayonnaise; med = medium; mg = milligram; na = not available; ord = order; oz = ounce; pkt = packet; reg = regular; Sat = saturated fat; sl = slice; sm = small; Tbsp = tablespoon; tr = trace; tsp = teaspoon; w/ = with; w/o = without

JACK-IN-THE-BOX

	Cal	Fat g	Sat g	Chol mg
BREAKFAST ITEMS				
Hash Browns (1 ord)	156	11	3	0
Breakfast Jack	307	13	5	20
Sourdough Breakfast Sandwich	381	20	7	236
Scrambled Egg Pocket	431	21	8	354
Pancake Platter	612	22	9	99
Scrambled Egg Platter	559	32	9	378
Crescent (1)				
Supreme	547	40	13	178
Sausage	584	43	16	187
SALADS				
Side	51	3	2	<1
Chef	325	18	8	142
Taco	503	31	13	92
FINGER FOODS				
Toasted Raviolis (10)	768	40	11	52
Egg Rolls (5)	753	41	12	49
Mini Chimichangas (6)	856	42	13	95
Chicken Wings (9)	1270	66	16	272
ENTRÉES				
Taco (1)	187	11	4	18
Super Taco (1)	281	17	6	29
HAMBURGERS				
Hamburger	267	11	4	26
Cheeseburger	315	14	6	41
Double	467	27	12	72
Bacon Bacon	705	45	15	113
Sharp Cheddar	886	59	na	92
Ultimate	942	69	26	127
Jumbo Jack	584	34	11	73
w/Cheese	677	40	14	102
Old Fashioned Patty Melt	713	46	15	92
Grilled Sourdough Burger	712	50	16	109

	Cal	Fat g	Sat g	Chol mg
SANDWICHES (1)				
Chicken Fajita Pita	292	8	3	34
Chicken & Mushroom	438	18	5	61
Grilled Chicken Fillet	431	19	5	65
Sirloin Steak	517	23	5	66
Country Fried Steak	450	25	7	36
Fish Supreme	510	27	6	55
Spicy Crispy Chicken	556	27	5	49
Smoked Chicken, Cheddar & Bacon	577	30	na	114
Beef Gyro	618	32	12	63
Chicken Supreme	641	39	10	85
SIDE ORDERS				
Sesame Breadsticks (1 ord)	70	2	na	0
Tortilla Chips (1 ord)	139	6	na	0
French Fries, sm	219	11	3	0
Reg	351	17	4	0
Jumbo	396	19	5	0
Seasoned Curly (1 ord)	358	20	5	0
Onion Rings (1 ord)	380	23	6	0
SAUCES AND CONDIMENTS				
Salsa (1 oz = 1 ord)	8	1	0	0
Guacamole (1 ord)	30	3	0	0
DESSERTS (1 ord)				
Double Fudge Cake	288	9	3	20
Cheesecake	309	18	9	63
Hot Apple Turnover	354	19	4	0
BEVERAGES				
Milk Shake				
Vanilla	320	6	4	25
Strawberry	320	7	4	25
Chocolate	330	7	4	25

c = cup; Cal = calories; Chol = cholesterol; diam = diameter; fl oz = fluid ounce; g = gram; lg = large; mayo = mayonnaise; med = medium; mg = milligram; na = not available; ord = order; oz = ounce; pkt = packet; reg = regular; Sat = saturated fat; sl = slice; sm = small; Tbsp = tablespoon; tr = trace; tsp = teaspoon; w/ = with; w/o = without

KENTUCKY FRIED CHICKEN

	Cal	Fat g	Sat g	Chol mg
ENTRÉES				
Kentucky Nuggets (1 nugget)	46	3	1	12
Original Recipe Chicken (1 piece)				
Drumstick	146	9	3	67
Wing	178	12	3	64
Center Breast	283	15	4	93
Side Breast	267	17	4	77
Thigh	294	20	5	123
Extra Tasty Crispy Chicken (1 piece)				
Drumstick	204	14	3	71
Wing	254	19	4	67
Center Breast	342	20	5	114
Side Breast	343	22	6	81
Thigh	406	30	8	129
Hot Wings (6)	376	24	5	148
SANDWICHES				
Chicken Littles	169	10	2	18
Colonel's Chicken	482	27	6	47
SAUCES				
Honey Sauce (½ oz)	49	0	0	0
Barbeque Sauce (1 oz)	35	1	0	0
Mustard Sauce (1 oz)	36	1	0	0
Sweet'n Sour Sauce (1 oz)	58	1	1	0
SIDE ORDERS				
Mashed Potatoes & Gravy (1 ord)	71	2	1	0
Corn-on-the-Cob (1 med)	176	3	1	0
Cole Slaw (1 ord)	119	7	1	5
Buttermilk Biscuit (1)	235	12	3	1
French Fries (1 ord)	244	12	3	2

LONG JOHN SILVER'S

	Cal	Fat g	Sat g	Chol mg
SALADS				
Side	25	1	0	0
Ocean Chef	110	1	0	40
Seafood	380	31	5	55
ENTRÉES				
Baked Lemon Crumb Fish (3 pieces)	150	1	0	110
Baked Light Herb Chicken (1 piece)	120	4	1	60
Baked Lemon Crumb Fish Dinner w/Rice & Side Salad (2 pieces)	330	5	1	75
Seafood Chowder w/Cod (7 oz)	140	6	2	20
Seafood Gumbo w/Cod (7 oz)	120	8	2	25
Batter-Dipped Chicken Sandwich w/o Sandwich Sauce (1 piece)	280	8	2	15
Batter-Dipped Fish Sandwich w/o Sandwich Sauce (1 piece)	340	13	3	30
Baked Lemon Crumb Fish Dinner w/Rice, Green Beans, Cole Slaw & Roll (3 pieces)	610	13	2	125
Baked Light Herb Chicken with Rice, Green Beans, Cole Slaw & Roll	590	15	3	75
Chicken Planks w/Fries (2 pieces)	490	26	6	30
Fish & Chicken Combination w/Fries (1 piece of each)	550	32	7	45
Fish & Fries (2 pieces)	610	37	8	60
Chicken Planks w/Fries, Cole Slaw & 2 Hushpuppies (3 pieces)	890	44	10	55

c = cup; Cal = calories; Chol = cholesterol; diam = diameter; fl oz = fluid ounce; g = gram; lg = large; mayo = mayonnaise; med = medium; mg = milligram; na = not available; ord = order; oz = ounce; pkt = packet; reg = regular; Sat = saturated fat; sl = slice; sm = small; Tbsp = tablespoon; tr = trace; tsp = teaspoon; w/ = with; w/o = without

	Cal	Fat g	Sat g	Chol mg
Entrées *(continued)*				
Shrimp w/Fries, Cole Slaw 2 Hushpuppies (10 shrimp)	840	47	10	100
Fish & More, Fries, Cole Slaw & Hushpuppies (2 pieces)	890	48	10	75
Fish & Chicken Combination w/Fries, Cole Slaw & 2 Hushpuppies (1 piece of fish, 2 pieces of Chicken)	950	49	11	75
Crispy Fish w/Fries, Cole Slaw & 2 Hushpuppies (3 Pieces)	980	50	11	70
Clams w/Fries, Cole Slaw & 2 Hushpuppies (6 oz clams)	990	52	11	75
Fish & Shrimp Combination w/Fries, Cole Slaw & 2 Hushpuppies (1 piece of fish, 8 shrimp)	1140	65	14	145
Fish, Shrimp & Chicken Combination w/Fries, Cole Slaw & 2 Hushpuppies (2 pieces of fish, 5 shrimp, 1 piece of chicken)	1160	65	14	135
Fish, Shrimp & Clams Combination w/Fries, Cole Slaw & 2 Hushpuppies (2 pieces of fish, 4 shrimp, 3 oz clams)	1240	70	15	140

KIDS' MEALS

	Cal	Fat g	Sat g	Chol mg
Fish & Fries w/1 Hushpuppy (1 piece)	500	28	6	30
Chicken Planks & Fries w/1 Hushpuppy (2 pieces)	560	29	6	30
Fish, Chicken & Fries w/1 Hushpuppy (1 piece of fish, 1 piece of chicken)	620	34	7	45

SIDE ORDERS

	Cal	Fat g	Sat g	Chol mg
Green Beans (1 ord)	20	1	0	0
Batter-Dipped Shrimp (1)	30	2	1	10
Hushpuppy (1)	70	2	1	<5
Rice (1 ord)	190	4	1	0

	Cal	Fat g	Sat g	Chol mg
Cole Slaw (drained on fork) (1 ord)	140	6	1	15
Corn Cobette (1)	140	8	na	0
Crispy Fish (1)	150	8	2	20
Batter-Dipped Fish (1 piece)	180	11	3	30
Chicken Planks (2)	240	12	3	3
French Fries (1 ord)	250	15	3	0

SAUCES

	Cal	Fat g	Sat g	Chol mg
Seafood Sauce (1 pkt)	14	1	0	0
Honey Mustard Sauce (1 pkt)	20	1	0	0
Sweet'n Sour Sauce (1 pkt)	20	1	0	0

DESSERTS

	Cal	Fat g	Sat g	Chol mg
Cookie (1)				
Chocolate Chip	230	9	6	10
Oatmeal Raisin	160	10	2	15
Pie (1 ord)				
Lemon	340	9	3	45
Apple	320	13	5	<5
Cherry	360	13	4	5
Walnut Brownie (1)	440	22	5	20

c = cup; Cal = calories; Chol = cholesterol; diam = diameter; fl oz = fluid ounce; g = gram; lg = large; mayo = mayonnaise; med = medium; mg = milligram; na = not available; ord = order; oz = ounce; pkt = packet; reg = regular; Sat = saturated fat; sl = slice; sm = small; Tbsp = tablespoon; tr = trace; tsp = teaspoon; w/ = with; w/o = without

McDONALD'S

	Cal	Fat g	Sat g	Chol mg
BREAKFAST ITEMS				
Fat-Free Apple Bran Muffin	180	0	0	0
English Muffin w/Spread	170	4	1	0
Hash Browns (1 ord)	130	7	1	0
Scrambled Eggs (2)	140	10	3	425
McMuffin, Egg	280	11	4	235
Sausage	345	20	7	57
Sausage w/Egg	430	25	8	270
Hotcakes w/Margarine (2 pats) & Syrup (1 ord)	440	12	2	8
Biscuit (1)				
w/Biscuit Spread	260	13	3	1
Bacon, Egg & Cheese	440	26	8	240
Sausage	420	28	8	44
Sausage w/Egg	505	33	10	260
Sausage (1 ord)	160	15	5	43
Danish (1)				
Raspberry	410	16	3	26
Apple	390	17	2	25
Iced Cheese	390	21	6	47
Cinnamon Raisin	440	21	5	34
Breakfast Burrito (1)	280	17	4	135
SALADS				
Side	30	1	0	33
Garden	50	2	0	65
Chunky Chicken	150	4	1	78
Chef	170	9	4	111
ENTRÉES				
Chicken Fajita (1)	190	8	2	35
Chicken McNuggets (9)	405	22	5	85
HAMBURGERS				
Hamburger	255	9	3	37
McLean Deluxe	320	10	4	60
w/Cheese	370	14	5	75
Cheeseburger	305	13	5	50

	Cal	Fat g	Sat g	Chol mg
Quarter Pounder	410	20	8	85
w/Cheese	510	28	11	115
Big Mac	500	26	9	100

SANDWICHES

	Cal	Fat g	Sat g	Chol mg
Filet-O-Fish	370	18	4	50
McChicken	415	20	4	50

SIDE ORDERS

	Cal	Fat g	Sat g	Chol mg
French Fries, sm	220	12	3	0
Med	320	17	4	0
Lg	400	22	5	0

SAUCES AND CONDIMENTS
(1 pkt)

	Cal	Fat g	Sat g	Chol mg
Honey	45	0	0	0
Bacon Bits	15	1	0	1
Barbeque Sauce	50	1	0	0
Sweet 'N Sour Sauce	60	1	0	0
Croutons	50	2	1	0
Hot Mustard Sauce	70	4	1	5

DESSERTS

	Cal	Fat g	Sat g	Chol mg
Vanilla Lowfat Frozen Yogurt Cone	105	1	0	3
Lowfat Frozen Yogurt Sundae				
Strawberry	210	1	0	5
Hot Fudge	240	3	2	6
Hot Caramel	270	3	2	13
McDonaldland Cookies (2 oz)	290	9	1	0
Baked Apple Pie (1 ord)	280	15	2	0
Chocolaty Chip Cookies (2 oz)	330	15	4	4

BEVERAGES

	Cal	Fat g	Sat g	Chol mg
Milk Shake				
Vanilla	310	5	3	25
Strawberry	340	5	3	25
Chocolate	350	6	4	25

c = cup; Cal = calories; Chol = cholesterol; diam = diameter; fl oz = fluid ounce; g = gram; lg = large; mayo = mayonnaise; med = medium; mg = milligram; na = not available; ord = order; oz = ounce; pkt = packet; reg = regular; Sat = saturated fat; sl = slice; sm = small; Tbsp = tablespoon; tr = trace; tsp = teaspoon; w/ = with; w/o = without

RAX

	Cal	Fat g	Sat g	Chol mg
SALADS				
Gourmet Garden	134	6	2	2
w/Lite Italian Dressing	196	10	2	2
w/French Dressing	409	29	5	2
Grilled Chicken Garden	202	9	2	32
w/Lite Italian Dressing	264	12	3	32
w/French Dressing	477	31	6	32
SANDWICHES				
Rax, reg	262	10	4	15
Philly Melt	396	16	7	27
Grilled Chicken Breast	402	23	4	69
Country Fried Chicken Breast	618	29	15	45
Deluxe Roast Beef	498	30	7	36
Beef, Bacon'n Cheddar	523	32	8	42
SIDE ORDERS				
Baked Potato	264	0	0	0
w/1 Tbsp Margarine	364	11	2	0
French Fries (1 ord)	282	14	4	3
SAUCES				
Cheddar Cheese (1 oz)	29	1	0	0
Mushroom (1 oz)	16	1	0	0
DESSERTS				
Chocolate Chip Cookie (2 oz)	262	12	4	6
BEVERAGES				
Colombo Fat Free Yogurt Shake				
Vanilla	220	0	0	0
Strawberry	300	0	0	0
Chocolate	310	0	0	0

	Cal	Fat g	Sat g	Chol mg
Colombo Yogurt Shake				
Blackberry	270	1	1	0
Candy Cane	320	4	3	0
Peach	320	4	3	0
Cool Orange	360	4	3	0
Mocha	350	7	5	0
Chocolate Chip	480	23	15	0
Chocolate Covered Cherry	540	23	15	0
Mint Chocolate Chip	570	23	15	0
Buckeye Peanut Butter Kiss	660	41	19	1

c = cup; Cal = calories; Chol = cholesterol; diam = diameter; fl oz = fluid ounce; g = gram; lg = large; mayo = mayonnaise; med = medium; mg = milligram; na = not available; ord = order; oz = ounce; pkt = packet; reg = regular; Sat = saturated fat; sl = slice; sm = small; Tbsp = tablespoon; tr = trace; tsp = teaspoon; w/ = with; w/o = without

RED LOBSTER

	Cal	Fat g	Sat g	Chol mg
APPETIZERS				
Shrimp Cocktail w/sauce (6 lg)	120	2	tr	175
Chilled Shrimp in Shell w/Sauce	160	2	1	250
Bayou Style Seafood Gumbo (6 oz)	180	5	1	38
12 oz	350	9	2	75
ENTRÉES				
Alaskan Snow Crab Legs (16 oz raw)	120	1	0	100
Live Maine Lobster (18 oz raw)	200	2	2	180
Broiled Rock Lobster (9 oz raw)	250	5	2	210
Skinless Chicken Breast (4 oz)	170	6	2	70
Grilled Shrimp Skewers (10 oz shrimp)	170	9	1	245
Atlantic Cod w/Butter Sauce (10 oz raw)	300	12	6	160
Broiled Flounder Fillets w/Butter Sauce (10 oz raw)	300	12	6	160
Grouper w/Butter Sauce (10 oz raw)	300	12	6	160
Haddock w/Butter Sauce (10 oz raw)	320	12	6	200
Lemon Sole w/Butter Sauce (10 oz raw)	320	12	6	150
Mahi Mahi w/Butter Sauce (10 oz raw)	320	12	6	206
Grilled Chicken Breast (8 oz)	340	12	4	140
Walleye Pike w/Butter Sauce (10 oz)	340	12	6	140
Yellow Lake Perch w/Butter Sauce (10 oz)	340	12	6	286
Sea Bass w/Butter Sauce (10 oz)	360	16	8	146
Swordfish w/Butter Sauce (10 oz)	300	18	12	600
Atlantic Ocean Perch w/Butter Sauce (10 oz)	360	18	10	170
Grilled Chicken & Shrimp (4 oz chicken & 10 shrimp)	490	20	6	300
Bay Platter (7 shrimp scampi, scallops, rice pilaf, 4 oz pollock)	500	20	7	280

	Cal	Fat g	Sat g	Chol mg
Shrimp Scampi (11)	310	23	14	290
Red Rock Fish w/Butter Sauce (10 oz raw)	560	24	12	380
Red Snapper w/Butter Sauce (10 oz)	640	24	12	340
Seafood Lover's Sampler (3 oz deviled crab, 7 shrimp, 2½ oz scallops, 4 oz pollock, 8 oz crab legs)	650	27	12	560
Rainbow Trout w/Butter Sauce (10 oz)	440	28	8	210
Coho Salmon w/Butter Sauce (10 oz)	480	28	10	138
Catfish w/Butter Sauce (10 oz)	440	30	12	200
Orange Roughy w/Butter Sauce (10 oz)	440	30	6	82
Atlantic Salmon w/Butter Sauce (10 oz)	460	34	12	158
King Salmon w/Butter Sauce (10 oz)	580	40	8	214

SANDWICHES

	Cal	Fat g	Sat g	Chol mg
Broiled Fish Fillet	300	10	tr	80
Grilled Chicken	340	10	4	70

SIDE ORDERS

	Cal	Fat g	Sat g	Chol mg
Fresh Vegetables (w/o butter sauce) (1 ord)	25	0	0	0
Baked Potato (oiled and salted) (1 ord)	270	2	tr	0
Lite Italian Dressing (1 oz)	50	3	tr	0
Rice Pilaf (1 ord)	140	3	tr	0
Shrimp Vinaigrette Dressing (1½ oz)	170	17	2	35

DESSERTS (1 ord)

	Cal	Fat g	Sat g	Chol mg
Sherbet	180	3	2	10
Ice Cream	260	14	9	60

c = cup; Cal = calories; Chol = cholesterol; diam = diameter; fl oz = fluid ounce; g = gram; lg = large; mayo = mayonnaise; med = medium; mg = milligram; na = not available; ord = order; oz = ounce; pkt = packet; reg = regular; Sat = saturated fat; sl = slice; sm = small; Tbsp = tablespoon; tr = trace; tsp = teaspoon; w/ = with; w/o = without

SHONEY'S

	Cal	Fat g	Sat g	Chol mg
BREAKFAST ITEMS				
Pancakes (1 6″ cake)	91	1	na	0
Breakfast Ham (2 sl)	59	2	na	28
Donut (1)				
Mini Cinnamon	56	3	na	0
Powdered Sugar	56	3	na	0
Grits (3 oz)	57	3	na	0
Hashbrowns (3 oz)	90	3	na	0
Home Fries (3 oz)	115	4	na	0
Jr. Bun (1)				
Chocolate	141	5	na	0
Honey	141	5	na	0
Maple	141	5	na	0
Brunch Cake (1 square)				
Pineapple	147	7	na	0
Carrot	150	7	na	0
Banana	152	7	na	0
Apple	160	8	na	0
Sour Cream	160	8	na	0
Blueberry Muffins (2)	214	7	na	33
Bacon Strips (3)	109	9	na	16
Country Gravy (3 oz)	114	10	na	2
Honey Bun (1)	265	14	na	3
Croissant (1)	260	16	na	2
Sirloin Steak, Charbroiled (6 oz)	357	25	na	99
SALADS				
Salad (¼ c)				
Ambrosia	75	3	na	0
Oriental	79	3	na	1
Pistachio Pineapple	98	3	na	0
Snow	72	4	na	0
Waldorf	81	5	na	2
ENTRÉES				
Boiled Shrimp	93	1	na	182
Baked Fish	170	1	na	83
Light Baked Fish	170	1	na	83

	Cal	Fat g	Sat g	Chol mg
Charbroiled Shrimp	138	3	na	162
Charbroiled Chicken	239	7	na	85
Hawaiian Chicken	262	7	na	85
Lasagna	297	10	na	26
Light Fried Fish	297	14	na	65
Spaghetti	496	16	na	55
Italian Feast	500	20	na	74
Shrimper's Feast	383	22	na	125
Lg	575	33	na	188
Light Beef Patty	289	23	na	82
Steak N'Shrimp (charbroiled)	361	23	na	141
Liver N'Onions	411	23	na	529
Shrimp Sampler	412	23	na	217
Sirloin (6 oz)	357	25	na	99
Bite Size Shrimp	387	25	na	140
Fish N'Shrimp	487	26	na	127
Country Fried Steak	449	27	na	27
Seafood Platter	566	28	na	127
Steak N'Shrimp (fried)	507	33	na	150
Half O Pound	435	34	na	123
Fish N'Chips	639	35	na	103
Ribeye (8 oz)	605	51	na	141

HAMBURGERS

	Cal	Fat g	Sat g	Chol mg
Old-Fashioned	470	28	na	82
All-American	501	33	na	86
Shoney	498	36	na	79
Bacon	591	40	na	86
Mushroom Swiss	616	42	na	106

SANDWICHES

	Cal	Fat g	Sat g	Chol mg
Baked Ham	290	10	na	42
Fish	323	13	na	21

c = cup; Cal = calories; Chol = cholesterol; diam = diameter; fl oz = fluid ounce; g = gram; lg = large; mayo = mayonnaise; med = medium; mg = milligram; na = not available; ord = order; oz = ounce; pkt = packet; reg = regular; Sat = saturated fat; sl = slice; sm = small; Tbsp = tablespoon; tr = trace; tsp = teaspoon; w/ = with; w/o = without

	Cal	Fat g	Sat g	Chol mg
Sandwiches *(continued)*				
Grilled Cheese	302	17	na	36
Charbroiled Chicken	451	17	na	90
Chicken Tenders	388	20	na	64
Chicken Fillet	464	21	na	51
Slim Jim	484	24	na	57
Country Fried	588	26	na	29
Grilled Bacon & Cheese	440	28	na	36
Club on Whole Wheat				
Turkey	635	33	na	100
Ham	642	36	na	78
Reuben	596	35	na	138
Patty Melt	640	42	na	121
Philly Steak Sandwich	673	44	na	103
SIDE ORDERS				
Onion Ring (1)	52	3	na	2
Sauteed Mushrooms (1 ord)	75	7	na	0
French Fries (4 oz)	252	10	na	0
DESSERTS (1 ord)				
Golden Pound Cake	134	5	na	13
Marble Cake w/Icing	136	5	na	0
Strawberry Pie	332	17	na	0
Strawberry Sundae	380	19	na	69
Hot Fudge Cake	522	20	na	27
Hot Fudge Sundae	451	22	na	60
Apple Pie A La Mode	492	23	na	35
Carrot Cake	500	26	na	37
Walnut Brownie A La Mode	576	34	na	35

SUBWAY

	Cal	Fat g	Sat g	Chol mg
SALADS				
Roast Beef, sm	222	10	4	38
Reg	340	20	7	75
Turkey Breast, sm	201	11	3	33
Reg	297	16	5	67
Ham & Cheese, sm	200	12	3	36
Reg	296	18	6	73
Club, sm	225	13	3	42
Reg	346	19	6	84
Veggies & Cheese, reg	188	14	4	19
Cold Cut Combo, sm	305	26	6	83
Reg	506	37	11	166
Seafood & Lobster, sm	351	28	5	28
Reg	597	49	9	55
BMT, sm	369	29	10	66
Reg	635	52	19	133
Seafood & Crab, sm	371	30	5	28
Reg	639	54	10	56
Spicy Italian, sm	400	33	12	68
Reg	696	60	22	137
Tuna, sm	430	38	7	43
Reg	755	68	12	85
SANDWICHES (12″ roll)				
Veggies & Cheese				
Italian Sub	535	17	6	19
Honey Wheat Sub	565	18	6	19
Ham & Cheese				
Italian Sub	653	18	7	73
Honey Wheat Sub	673	22	7	73
Turkey Breast				
Italian Sub	645	19	6	67
Honey Wheat Sub	674	20	6	67

c = cup; Cal = calories; Chol = cholesterol; diam = diameter; fl oz = fluid ounce; g = gram; lg = large; mayo = mayonnaise; med = medium; mg = milligram; na = not available; ord = order; oz = ounce; pkt = packet; reg = regular; Sat = saturated fat; sl = slice; sm = small; Tbsp = tablespoon; tr = trace; tsp = teaspoon; w/ = with; w/o = without

	Cal	Fat g	Sat g	Chol mg
Sandwiches *(continued)*				
Subway Club				
Italian Sub	693	22	7	84
Honey Wheat Sub	722	23	7	84
Roast Beef				
Italian Sub	689	23	8	75
Honey Wheat Sub	717	24	8	75
Steak & Cheese				
Italian Sub	765	32	12	82
Honey Wheat Sub	711	33	12	82
Cold Cut Combo				
Italian Sub	853	40	12	166
Honey Wheat Sub	883	41	12	166
Meatball				
Italian Sub	918	44	17	88
Honey Wheat Sub	947	45	17	88
Seafood & Lobster				
Italian Sub	944	53	11	55
Honey Wheat Sub	974	54	11	55
BMT				
Italian Sub	982	55	20	133
Honey Wheat Sub	1011	57	20	133
Seafood & Crab				
Italian Sub	986	57	11	56
Honey Wheat Sub	1015	58	11	56
Spicy Italian				
Italian Sub	1043	63	23	137
Honey Wheat Sub	1073	64	23	137
Tuna				
Italian Sub	1103	72	13	85
Honey Wheat Sub	1132	73	10	85
DESSERTS				
Cookies (1½ oz)				
Chocolate Candy	192	8	na	na
White Chocolate Chip w/Macadamia Nuts & Almonds	204	9	na	na
Milk Chocolate Chip	195	10	na	na

TACO BELL

	Cal	Fat g	Sat g	Chol mg
SALADS				
Taco Salad w/o shell	484	31	14	80
w/shell	905	61	19	80
ENTRÉES				
Pintos 'N Cheese w/Red Sauce (1 ord)	190	9	4	16
Burrito (1)				
Fiesta Bean w/Red Sauce	226	9	3	9
Chicken	334	12	4	52
Bean w/Red Sauce	447	14	4	9
Combination w/Red Sauce	407	16	5	33
Beef w/Red Sauce	493	21	8	57
Supreme w/Red Sauce	503	22	8	33
Taco (1)	183	11	5	32
Fiesta	127	7	3	16
Supreme	230	15	8	32
BellGrande	335	23	11	56
Tostada w/Red Sauce (1)	243	11	4	16
Soft Taco (1)	225	12	5	32
Fiesta	147	7	3	16
Chicken	213	10	4	52
Steak	218	11	5	30
Supreme	272	16	8	32
MexiMelt (1)				
Chicken	257	15	7	48
Beef	266	15	8	38
Chilito (1)	383	18	8	47
Enchirito w/Red Sauce (1)	382	20	9	54
Mexican Pizza	575	37	11	52
SIDE ORDERS				
Cinnamon Twists (1 ord)	171	8	3	0
Nachos (1 ord)	346	18	6	9
Supreme	376	27	5	18
BellGrande	649	35	12	36

c = cup; Cal = calories; Chol = cholesterol; diam = diameter; fl oz = fluid ounce; g = gram; lg = large; mayo = mayonnaise; med = medium; mg = milligram; na = not available; ord = order; oz = ounce; pkt = packet; reg = regular; Sat = saturated fat; sl = slice; sm = small; Tbsp = tablespoon; tr = trace; tsp = teaspoon; w/ = with; w/o = without

TACO JOHN'S INTERNATIONAL

	Cal	Fat g	Sat g	Chol mg
SALADS				
Taco	228	13	na	na
w/Dressing	359	24	na	na
Chicken Super Taco	377	15	na	na
w/Dressing	507	27	na	na
Super Taco	428	20	na	na
w/Dressing	558	32	na	na
ENTRÉES				
Burrito (1)				
Bean	197	6	na	na
Chicken	227	10	na	na
Combo	250	12	na	na
Super w/Chicken	366	14	na	na
Chicken w/Green Chili	344	16	na	na
Super	389	17	na	na
Beef	303	18	na	na
Smothered w/Green Chili	367	18	na	na
Smothered w/Texas Chili	455	23	na	na
Taco (1)	178	13	na	na
w/Chicken	140	9	na	na
Softshell Taco (1)	224	13	na	na
w/Chicken	180	8	na	na
Taco Burger	281	14	na	na
Taco Bravo (1)	319	14	na	na
Super	361	19	na	na
Chimichanga (1)	464	21	na	na
w/Chicken	441	19	na	na
SIDE ORDERS				
Mexican Rice (1 ord)	340	8	na	na
Larger Potato Ole (1 ord)	414	24	na	na
Nachos (1 ord)	468	25	na	na
Super	669	39	na	na

WENDY'S

	Cal	Fat g	Sat g	Chol mg
SALADS				
Side	60	3	0	0
Deluxe Garden	110	5	1	0
Caesar Side	160	6	1	10
Grilled Chicken	200	8	1	55
Taco	640	30	12	80
ENTRÉES				
Baked Potato, plain	300	1	0	0
w/Sour Cream & Chives	370	6	4	15
w/Broccoli & Cheese	450	14	2	0
w/Bacon & Cheese	510	17	4	15
w/Cheese	550	24	8	30
w/Chili & Cheese	600	25	9	45
Chili (1 lg)	290	9	4	60
Crispy Chicken Nuggets (6)	280	20	5	50
HAMBURGERS				
Hamburger				
Jr. & Kids' Meal	270	9	3	35
¼-lb Hamburger Patty	190	12	5	70
Plain Single	350	15	6	70
Single w/Everything	440	23	7	75
Cheeseburger				
Kids' Meal	310	13	5	45
Jr.	320	13	5	45
Jr. Deluxe	390	20	7	50
Jr. Bacon	440	25	8	65
Big Classic	480	23	7	75
SANDWICHES				
Grilled Chicken	290	7	1	60
Breaded Chicken	450	20	4	60

c = cup; Cal = calories; Chol = cholesterol; diam = diameter; fl oz = fluid ounce; g = gram; lg = large; mayo = mayonnaise; med = medium; mg = milligram; na = not available; ord = order; oz = ounce; pkt = packet; reg = regular; Sat = saturated fat; sl = slice; sm = small; Tbsp = tablespoon; tr = trace; tsp = teaspoon; w/ = with; w/o = without

	Cal	Fat g	Sat g	Chol mg
Sandwiches *(continued)*				
Fish	460	25	5	55
Chicken Club	520	25	6	75
Country Fried Steak	460	26	7	35

SIDE ORDERS

	Cal	Fat g	Sat g	Chol mg
French Fries, sm	240	12	2	0
Med	360	17	4	0
Biggie	450	22	5	0

DESSERTS

	Cal	Fat g	Sat g	Chol mg
Strawberry Banana Dessert (¼ c)	110	1	0	0
Pudding (¼ c), Chocolate & Vanilla	80	3	na	0
Frosty Dairy Dessert, sm	340	10	5	40
Med	460	13	7	55
Lg	570	17	9	70
Chocolate Chip Cookie (1)	280	13	4	15

WHITE CASTLE

	Cal	Fat g	Sat g	Chol mg
HAMBURGERS				
Hamburger	161	8	na	na
Cheeseburger	200	11	na	na
SANDWICHES				
Fish w/o Tartar Sauce	155	5	na	na
Chicken	186	8	na	na
Sausage	196	12	na	na
w/Egg	322	22	na	na
SIDE ORDERS (1 ord)				
Onion Rings	245	13	na	na
French Fries	301	15	na	na
Onion Chips	329	17	na	na

c = cup; Cal = calories; Chol = cholesterol; diam = diameter; fl oz = fluid ounce; g = gram; lg = large; mayo = mayonnaise; med = medium; mg = milligram; na = not available; ord = order; oz = ounce; pkt = packet; reg = regular; Sat = saturated fat; sl = slice; sm = small; Tbsp = tablespoon; tr = trace; tsp = teaspoon; w/ = with; w/o = without

Chapter 5

Airline and Cruise Ship Cuisine

People traveling by air have the opportunity to dine on the type of food they prefer. Most airlines now offer a number of special meals in both coach and first-class cabins. These meals are designed to take health needs, religious requirements, and lifestyle preferences into consideration. The meals designed for "health needs" include low-fat, low-sodium, diabetic, and lactose-free. Those meals provided to fulfill "religious requirements" include kosher, Moslem, and Hindu. Meals designated for "lifestyle" preferences include vegetarian, fruit plate, or seafood (hot or cold). Most of these meals are available, on prior request, for breakfast, lunch, or dinner. The special meals that are usually lowest in fat and saturated fat are "low-fat," "low-cholesterol," "low-calorie," and "diabetic." The following table shows the special meals available on each airline.

The best time to request a special meal is when you make your reservation. However, if it is necessary for you to change your flight schedule, your special meal probably will not make the change with you.

Regular airline meals traditionally have been high in fat and sodium, and, except for the special meals, the airlines have offered no choices. Now airlines offer more choices, such as between a beef and a chicken entrée; at times a meatless entrée, such as pasta, may be offered. Some airlines offer popular foods such as pizza, hamburgers, and frozen desserts; however, these foods are higher in fat than the lower-fat special meals listed above. Some foreign airlines offer ethnic foods, such as Oriental meals, and some domestic airlines are combining ethnic entrées, such as Mexican, with traditional salads and desserts.

More commercially packaged foods—bread, cookies, yogurt, salad dressings, crackers, and margarine—are appearing on airline trays. Some airlines have the foods repackaged in clear cellophane, while others leave the manufacturer's name on them.

Peanuts are the most common and most popular snack food served on planes: however, some airlines now serve pretzels, which are lower in fat. A small package (½ ounce) of peanuts provides the following:

	Cal	Fat g	Sat g	Chol mg
Peanuts, dry roasted & oil-roasted	82	7	1	0
Peanuts, honey-roasted	77	6	1	0

	AA	AC	AP	AU	CO	CP	DL	LA	LU	LY	NW	NZ	QF	UA	US
Asian vegetarian			✓			✓	✓	✓	✓				✓	✓	
Baby			✓			✓	✓	✓			✓	✓	✓	✓	
Bland or soft	✓		✓	✓	✓	✓	✓	✓	✓		✓	✓	✓		✓
Child or toddler	✓		✓	✓	✓	✓	✓	✓			✓	✓	✓	✓	✓
Dairy										✓					
Diabetic	✓		✓	✓	✓	✓	✓	✓	✓	✓	✓	✓	✓	✓	✓
Fasting—Ethiopian Lent										✓					
Fasting—Greek Orthodox Lent										✓					
Fish		✓							✓	✓	✓				
Fluid or semifluid													✓		
Fruit plate		✓					✓				✓	✓	✓		
Gluten-free or lactose-free	✓		✓	✓		✓	✓	✓	✓		✓	✓	✓	✓	
High-fiber			✓	✓		✓		✓	✓			✓	✓		
High-protein					✓										✓
Hindu	✓	✓	✓		✓	✓		✓	✓		✓	✓	✓	✓	✓
Kosher	✓	✓	✓		✓	✓		✓			✓	✓	✓	✓	✓
Low-calorie	✓	✓	✓		✓	✓		✓	✓			✓	✓	✓	✓
Low-carbohydrate	✓					✓					✓		✓	✓	
Low-fat/low-cholesterol	✓	✓	✓	✓	✓	✓	✓	✓	✓		✓	✓	✓	✓	✓

	AA	AC	AP	AU	CO	CP	DL	LA	LU	LY	NW	NZ	QF	UA	US
Low-protein			✓	✓				✓					✓		
Low-purine			✓	✓		✓		✓	✓			✓			
Low-sodium	✓		✓	✓	✓	✓	✓	✓	✓	✓	✓	✓	✓	✓	✓
Medical pre-cut													✓		
Mormon													✓		
Moslem meal	✓		✓		✓	✓	✓	✓	✓		✓	✓	✓	✓	✓
Oriental	✓					✓						✓			
Parve—no meat or dairy										✓					
Raw vegetarian				✓		✓			✓			✓			
Refugee											✓				
Seafood—cold							✓				✓			✓	✓
Seafood—hot			✓	✓		✓	✓					✓	✓	✓	✓
Sulfite-free											✓				
Vegetarian—Indian													✓		
Vegetarian—ovolacto	✓		✓		✓	✓	✓	✓			✓	✓	✓		✓
Vegetarian—pure	✓	✓	✓	✓	✓	✓	✓	✓	✓	✓	✓	✓	✓		
White meat												✓	✓		

AA = American Airlines; AC = Air Canada; AP = Air Portugal; AU = Austrian Airlines; CO = Continental Airlines; CP = Canadian Airlines; DL = Delta Air Lines; LA = Ladeco Airlines of Chile; LU = Lufthansa; LY = El Al Israel Airlines; NW = Northwest Airlines; NZ = Air New Zealand; QF = Qantas Airways; UA = United Airlines; US = USAir

Passengers on cruise ships can choose from an abundance of food, often made available morning, noon, night, and in between. The dinner menu on a cruise ship typically offers a number of courses, including appetizer, soup, salad, pasta, main course, and dessert. Some cruise ship menus indicate foods that are low in cholesterol; these dishes may *not* be low in fat and/or saturated fat. It takes some planning and self-control to select reasonable amounts of foods that are lower in fat from among the numerous dishes being offered. The tips on selecting foods lower in fat and sodium that are listed throughout this book also apply to cruise ship cuisine.

TRAVELING AND JET LAG

Anyone who travels long distances by air may suffer the effects of jet lag. Jet lag may be recognized as fatigue, sleepiness, inability to sleep, gastrointestinal upset, and/or decreased mental activity. It is a disturbance of the body's normal cycle of sleeping and waking—the biological clock—that is caused by flying across time zones.

One of the authors (Dr. DeBakey) has logged millions of miles by air during visits to most countries of the world. Since these trips usually require attending medical meetings, lecturing, holding conferences, or performing or demonstrating surgical procedures, his ability to minimize jet lag is essential. To decrease the risk of gastrointestinal upsets, Dr. DeBakey emphasizes the importance of carefully selecting what you eat (see list on page 143).

DR. DeBAKEY'S TIPS ON TRAVELING

Decreasing Jet Lag
- **Sleep as much as possible on the airplane—ask that the steward or stewardess not awaken you for meals. Sleeping is much more important than reading, studying, or writing.**

Dr. DeBakey's Tips on Traveling
(*continued*)

- Eat a light meal before boarding the air-plane, since a heavy meal tends to increase fatigue and to interfere with sleep.
- During the flight, drink plenty of fluids that do not have caffeine or alcohol. Although some travelers think that alcohol has a tranquilizing effect, the ultimate result is increased fatigue and a depression of mental activity.
- Assume the local schedule of eating and sleeping as soon as you reach your destination. Being outdoors in the sunlight helps you adjust to the new light/dark cycle.

Decreasing the Risk of Gastrointestinal Upset in Foreign Countries

- Eat only foods that are cooked. Raw foods washed in the local water may carry bacteria that will cause diarrhea or nausea. Avoid all raw vegetables and fruits, except fruits that can be peeled, such as bananas and oranges.
- Drink only bottled water. This includes the water used to take medications and to brush your teeth.

ESTIMATING YOUR CALORIE LEVEL

Follow these four steps to estimate your calorie level:

1. *Height*—measured without shoes.

2. *Frame size*—calculated by using wrist size. Use one of two simple methods to determine your frame size. In the first method, place the thumb and index finger of one hand around your other wrist, making sure your thumb and index finger go around the radius and ulna bones at your wrist (the smallest part, closest to your hand).

- If thumb and index finger *overlap,* you have a *small* frame.
- If thumb and index finger *just touch,* you have a *medium* frame.
- If thumb and index finger *do not meet,* you have a *large* frame.

The second way to determine frame size requires a flexible measuring tape, which is used to measure around your wrist at the smallest area, nearest your hand. Match your wrist measurement with your height in the table below to get your frame size.

Height	Small Frame	Medium Frame	Large Frame
Under 5'3"	Less than 5½"	5½" to 5¾"	Greater than 5¾"
5'3" to 5'4"	Less than 6"	6" to 6¼"	Greater than 6¼"
Over 5'4"	Less than 6¼"	6¼" to 6½"	Greater than 6½"

3. *Activity level*—based on all of your activities for a typical day. Consider the amount of time you spend resting, walking around your house, sitting at a desk, watching television, and exercising to determine your level of activity from the list below.

ADULT MALES

Height Without Shoes	Frame Size	Desirable Weight (Pounds)	Calorie Level Based on Physical Activity				
			Very Light (Calories)	Light (Calories)	Moderate (Calories)	Heavy (Calories)	
5'5"	Small	129 (124–133)	1,700	1,950	2,200	2,600
	Medium	137 (130–143)	1,800	2,050	2,350	2,750
	Large	147 (138–156)	1,900	2,200	2,500	2,950
5'6"	Small	133 (128–137)	1,750	2,000	2,250	2,650
	Medium	141 (134–147)	1,850	2,100	2,400	2,800
	Large	152 (142–161)	2,000	2,300	2,600	3,050
5'7"	Small	137 (132–141)	1,800	2,050	2,350	2,750
	Medium	145 (138–152)	1,900	2,200	2,450	2,900
	Large	157 (147–166)	2,050	2,350	2,650	3,150
5'8"	Small	141 (136–145)	1,850	2,100	2,400	2,850
	Medium	149 (142–156)	1,950	2,250	2,550	3,000
	Large	161 (151–170)	2,100	2,400	2,750	3,200
5'9"	Small	145 (140–150)	1,900	2,200	2,450	2,900
	Medium	153 (146–160)	2,000	2,300	2,600	3,050
	Large	165 (155–174)	2,150	2,500	2,800	3,300
5'10"	Small	149 (144–154)	1,950	2,250	2,550	3,000
	Medium	158 (150–165)	2,050	2,350	2,700	3,150
	Large	169 (159–179)	2,200	2,550	2,850	3,400

Calorie Level Based on Physical Activity

Height Without Shoes	Frame Size	Desirable Weight (Pounds)	Very Light (Calories)	Light (Calories)	Moderate (Calories)	Heavy (Calories)
5'11"	Small	153 (148–158)	2,000	2,300	2,600	3,050
	Medium	162 (154–170)	2,100	2,450	2,750	3,250
	Large	174 (164–184)	2,250	2,600	2,950	3,500
6'0"	Small	157 (152–162)	2,050	2,350	2,650	3,150
	Medium	167 (158–175)	2,150	2,500	2,850	3,350
	Large	179 (168–189)	2,350	2,700	3,050	3,600
6'1"	Small	162 (156–167)	2,100	2,450	2,750	3,250
	Medium	171 (162–180)	2,200	2,550	2,900	3,400
	Large	184 (173–194)	2,400	2,750	3,150	3,700
6'2"	Small	166 (160–171)	2,150	2,500	2,800	3,300
	Medium	176 (167–185)	2,300	2,650	3,000	3,500
	Large	189 (178–199)	2,450	2,850	3,200	3,800
6'3"	Small	170 (164–175)	2,200	2,550	2,900	3,400
	Medium	181 (172–190)	2,350	2,700	3,100	3,600
	Large	193 (182–204)	2,500	2,900	3,300	3,850

Adapted from 1959 Metropolitan Life Insurance Company, New York City. These tables are based on 1959 rather than 1983 Metropolitan Life Insurance Company height-weight tables because the earlier tables specify lower weights, more appropriate to health-related concerns.

ADULT FEMALES

Height Without Shoes	Frame Size	Desirable Weight (Pounds)	Calorie Level Based on Physical Activity			
			Very Light (Calories)	Light (Calories)	Moderate (Calories)	Heavy (Calories)
5'0"	Small	106 (102–110)	1,400	1,600	1,800	2,100
	Medium	113 (107–119)	1,450	1,700	1,900	2,250
	Large	123 (115–131)	1,600	1,850	2,100	2,450
5'1"	Small	109 (105–113)	1,400	1,650	1,850	2,200
	Medium	116 (110–122)	1,500	1,750	1,950	2,300
	Large	126 (118–134)	1,650	1,900	2,150	2,500
5'2"	Small	112 (108–116)	1,450	1,700	1,900	2,250
	Medium	119 (113–126)	1,550	1,800	2,000	2,400
	Large	129 (121–138)	1,700	1,950	2,200	2,600
5'3"	Small	115 (111–119)	1,500	1,750	1,950	2,300
	Medium	123 (116–130)	1,600	1,850	2,100	2,450
	Large	133 (125–142)	1,750	2,000	2,250	2,650
5'4"	Small	118 (114–123)	1,550	1,750	2,000	2,350
	Medium	127 (120–135)	1,650	1,900	2,150	2,550
	Large	137 (129–146)	1,800	2,050	2,350	2,750
5'5"	Small	122 (118–127)	1,600	1,850	2,050	2,450
	Medium	131 (124–139)	1,700	1,950	2,250	2,600
	Large	141 (133–150)	1,850	2,100	2,400	2,800

Calorie Level Based on Physical Activity

Height Without Shoes	Frame Size	Desirable Weight (Pounds)	Very Light (Calories)	Light (Calories)	Moderate (Calories)	Heavy (Calories)
5'6"	Small	126 (122–131)	1,650	1,900	2,150	2,500
	Medium	135 (128–143)	1,750	2,050	2,300	2,700
	Large	145 (137–154)	1,900	2,200	2,450	2,900
5'7"	Small	130 (126–135)	1,700	1,950	2,200	2,600
	Medium	139 (132–147)	1,800	2,100	2,350	2,800
	Large	149 (141–158)	1,950	2,250	2,550	3,000
5'8"	Small	135 (130–140)	1,750	2,050	2,300	2,700
	Medium	143 (136–151)	1,850	2,150	2,450	2,850
	Large	154 (145–163)	2,000	2,300	2,600	3,100
5'9"	Small	139 (134–144)	1,800	2,100	2,350	2,800
	Medium	147 (140–155)	1,900	2,200	2,500	2,950
	Large	158 (149–168)	2,050	2,350	2,700	3,150
5'10"	Small	143 (138–148)	1,850	2,150	2,450	2,850
	Medium	151 (144–159)	1,950	2,250	2,550	3,000
	Large	163 (153–173)	2,100	2,450	2,750	3,250

Adapted from 1959 Metropolitan Life Insurance Company, New York City. These tables are based on 1959 rather than 1983 Metropolitan Life Insurance Company height-weight tables because the earlier tables specify lower weights, more appropriate to health-related concerns.

ACTIVITY LEVEL

- *Very Light Activity*
  Seated and standing activities, such as working in a laboratory, driving, typing, sewing, ironing, cooking, playing cards, playing a musical instrument.
- *Light Activity*
  Walking on a level surface at 2.5 to 3 mph, garage work, electrical work, restaurant work, carpentry, housecleaning, child care, golf, sailing, table tennis.
- *Moderate Activity*
  Walking 3.5 to 4 mph, weeding, carrying a load, cycling, skiing, tennis, dancing.
- *Heavy Activity*
  Walking uphill with a load, heavy manual labor such as digging, climbing, basketball, football, soccer.

Adapted from National Research Council, *Recommended Dietary Allowance,* 10th Edition. National Academy Press, Washington, D.C., 1989.

4. *Calorie level*—calculated by finding your height, frame size, and level of activity in the following table either for males or for females. The daily calorie levels in these tables are estimates only and are based on ideal body weight. Each person is an individual, and you may actually need a higher or lower calorie level than that shown in the table. For example, you will need to add calories if you wish to gain weight or during pregnancy or lactation. If you are overweight, the calorie levels in the tables are probably lower than what you typically consume each day. Overestimating your physical activity can cause the calorie level given in the table to be too high. For example, if you consider yourself moderately active, but you actually do mostly light physical activity, the calorie level indicated in the table will be too high for you. Very few people do heavy physical activity on a regular basis.

CALCULATING GRAMS OF FAT AND SATURATED FAT

To calculate your maximum recommended number of grams of fat and saturated fat, find your calorie level in the table below. The grams of fat in the table represent

30% of calories at each calorie level; the grams of saturated fat represent 10% of calories.

CALORIE LEVELS: GRAMS OF FAT AND SATURATED FAT

Calorie Level	Fat* (g)	Saturated Fat* (g)
1,200	40	13
1,300	43	14
1,400	47	16
1,500	50	17
1,600	53	18
1,700	57	19
1,800	60	20
1,900	63	21
2,000	67	22
2,100	70	23
2,200	73	24
2,300	77	26
2,400	80	27
2,500	83	28
2,600	87	29
2,700	90	30
2,800	93	31
2,900	97	32
3,000	100	33

*Grams of fat equal to 30% of calories and grams of saturated fat equal to 10% of calories.

If your calorie level does not appear in the previous table, you can estimate the grams of fat and grams of saturated fat for your calorie level using the following formula. For example, to determine maximum recommended grams of fat (30% of calories) and saturated fat (10% of calories) at the 2,250-calorie level:

1. Multiply calorie level (2,250) by .3 (30%) = 675 calories from fat.

2. Divide calories from fat (675) by 9 (calories in 1 gram of fat) = 75 grams of fat (equal to 30% of 2,250 calories from fat).

3. Divide the grams of fat representing 30% of 2,250 calories (75) by 3 = 25 grams of saturated fat (grams of saturated fatty acids equal to 10%, or one third of 30%, of 2,250 calories).

Therefore, at an intake of 2,250 calories, a *maximum* of 75 grams of fat and less than 25 grams of saturated fat is recommended each day. If you eat a food high in fat, you will need to select lower-fat foods during the rest of the day to compensate for it.

Ballas B., Catsinas H., Glaros C., Harrison S., eds. *Greek Gourmet Cooking*. Privately printed: Socrates Payavla and Pete Verges, 1973.

Best Recipes from Time-Life Books. New York: Wings Books, 1986.

Bettoja J., Cornetto A. M. *Italian Cooking in the Grand Tradition*. New York: Simon & Schuster, 1982.

Bocuse P. *Bocuse's Regional French Cooking*. Translated by S. Curtis. Flammarion.

Cecconi A. *Betty Crocker's Italian Cooking*. New York: Prentice Hall Press, 1991.

Cheng R., Morris M. *Chinese Cookery*. Tucson: HP Books, Inc., 1981.

Child J. *The French Chef Cookbook*. New York: Bantam Books, 1981.

Conte A. D. *The Italian Pantry*. New York: Harper & Row, 1990.

Culinary Institute of America. *The New Professional Chef,* fifth edition, Conway L. G., ed. New York: Van Nostrand Reinhold, 1991.

de Boos-Smith F. *The Best of Italian Cooking*. London: Bay Books, 1984.

DeMers J. *Arnaud's Creole Cookbook*. New York: Simon & Schuster, 1988.

Downer L., Yoneda M. *Step by Step Japanese Cooking*. London: Quarto Publishing, Ltd., 1986.

Fuermann G. *Tony's The Cookbook*. Fredericksburg, Tex.: Shearer Publishing Ltd., 1986.

Gisslen W. *Professional Cooking,* second edition. New York: John Wiley & Sons, 1989.

Greek Festival, Annunciation Greek Orthodox Cathedral, *Greek Gourmet Cooking*. Privately printed: Carl Gren Lithographing and Printing, 1976.

Hazan M. *Essentials of Classic Italian Cooking*. New York: Alfred A. Knopf, 1992.

Huang D. *Dorothy Huang's Chinese Cooking*. Houston: Pinewood Press, 1980.

Kochilas D. *The Food and Wine of Greece*. New York: St. Martin's Press, 1990.

Mallos T. *The Complete Middle East Cookbook*. Chicago: Weldon Publishing, 1979.

Minnesota Nutrition Data System software, developed by the Nutrition Coordinating Center, University of Minnesota, Minneapolis. Food Database Version 6A: Nutrient Database version 21.

O'Connell R. M. *365 Easy Italian Recipes*. New York: HarperCollins Publishers, 1991.

Orsini J. *Father Orsini's Italian Kitchen*. New York: St. Martin's Press, 1991.

Passmore J. *The Encyclopedia of Asian Food and Cooking*. New York: William Morrow and Company, 1991.

Pépin J. *La Technique Jacques Pépin*. New York: Pocket Books, 1978.

Poladitmontri P., Lew J. *Thailand The Beautiful Cookbook*. San Francisco: Collins Publishers, 1992.

Prudhomme P. *Chef Paul Prudhomme's Louisiana Kitchen*. New York: William Morrow and Company, 1984.

Quintana P. *The Taste of Mexico*. New York: Stewart, Tabori & Chang, 1986.

Recipes: The Cooking of Japan. New York: Time-Life Books, 1969.

Routhier N. *The Foods of Vietnam*. New York: Stewart, Tabori & Chang, 1989.

Salah N. *One Thousand and One Delights*. Published and distributed by Nahda Salah, n.d.

Shugart G., Molt M. *Food For Fifty,* ninth edition. New York: Macmillan Publishing Company, 1993.

Stendahl. *The Bombay Palace Cookbook*. New York: Caravan Publishing, 1985.

USDA Agriculture Handbook No. 8 series.

Warner J. *A Taste of Chinatown*. Toronto: Flavor Publications, 1989.

Michael E. DeBakey, M.D., is one of the most eminent heart surgeons in the world. He was among the first to complete a successful heart transplant in the United States and has pioneered new methods for the diagnosis and treatment of heart disease. Among Dr. DeBakey's numerous noted surgical accomplishments are the first successful resection and graft replacement of an aneurysm of the thoracic aorta and first successful coronary artery bypass. Currently, he is Chancellor of Baylor College of Medicine, Distinguished Service Professor of its Department of Surgery, and Director of The DeBakey Heart Center.

Antonio M. Gotto, Jr., M.D., D.Phil., is one of the world's most important specialists in research on fats in the blood and their role in the development of coronary heart disease. He serves as the Principal Investigator of the Baylor College of Medicine Specialized Center of Research in Atherosclerosis of the National Institutes of Health. Currently, he serves as the Chairman of the Department of Medicine at Baylor College of Medicine and Chief of Internal Medicine Service at The Methodist Hospital, both of Houston, Texas.

Lynne W. Scott, M.A., R.D./L.D., is Assistant Professor in the Department of Medicine and Director of the Diet Modification Clinic at Baylor College of Medicine and The Methodist Hospital. She serves as a member of the National Cholesterol Education Program Expert Panel on Blood Cholesterol Levels in Children and Adolescents. She is a registered dietitian and clinical researcher investigating the effect of dietary components on blood cholesterol. She has 42 publications in the area of nutrition and serves on several nutrition committees of the national American Heart Association.

Mary Carole McMann, M.P.H., R.D./L.D., is a research dietitian and a nutrition counselor in the Diet Modification Clinic at Baylor College of Medicine and

The Methodist Hospital. She is a contributing author of *The Living Heart Brand Name Shopper's Guide* and "A Look at Eating Habits and Heart Disease Around the World," published in the *Encyclopaedia Britannica 1993 Medical and Health Annual*; is Associate Editor of *Panic in the Pantry* (1992); and has written numerous magazine, newsletter, and newspaper articles on health-related subjects.

Suzanne M. Jaax, M.S., R.D./L.D., is a research dietitian in the Diet Modification Clinic at Baylor College of Medicine and The Methodist Hospital. She is involved in research on cholesterol, including the nutrition component of a study investigating regression in coronary atherosclerosis. She is also involved in a study investigating the effect of very-low-fat diets on skin cancer. She is a contributing author of *The Living Heart Brand Name Shopper's Guide*.

Danièle Brauchi, R.D./L.D., is a research dietitian and a nutrition counselor at the Diet Modification Clinic at Baylor College of Medicine and The Methodist Hospital. She specializes in the dietary treatment of hyperlipidemia and is a contributing author of *The Living Heart Brand Name Shopper's Guide*. She is a native of France and completed her degree and nutrition training in the United States.

To order MasterMedia books, either go to your local bookstore or call (800) 334-8232.

HEALTH, FITNESS, BEAUTY

THE LIVING HEART BRAND NAME SHOPPER'S GUIDE (Revised and Updated), by Michael E. DeBakey, M.D., Antonio M. Gotto, Jr., M.D., D.Phil., Lynne W. Scott, M.A., R.D./L.D., and John P. Foreyt, Ph.D. ($14.95 paper)

PAIN RELIEF! How to Say No to Acute, Chronic, and Cancer Pain, by Jane Cowles, Ph.D. ($22.95 cloth)

STRAIGHT TALK ON WOMEN'S HEALTH: How to Get the Health Care You Deserve, by Janice Teal, Ph.D., and Phyllis Schneider ($14.95 paper)

YOUR HEALTHY BODY, YOUR HEALTHY LIFE: How to Take Control of Your Medical Destiny, by Donald B. Louria, M.D. ($12.95 paper)

REAL BEAUTY . . . REAL WOMEN: A Handbook for Making the Best of Your Own Good Looks, by Kathleen Walas, International Beauty and Fashion Director of Avon Products ($19.50 paper; in full color)

THE OUTDOOR WOMAN: A Handbook to Adventure, by Patricia Hubbard and Stan Wass ($14.95 paper; with photos)

MANAGING ATTENTION DEFICIT DISORDER IN YOUR FAMILY, by Bill Cooper ($11.95 paper, $19.95 cloth)

THE LIVING HEART GUIDE TO EATING OUT, by Michael E. DeBakey, M.D., Antonio M. Gotto, Jr., M.D., D.Phil., and Lynne W. Scott, M.A., R.D./L.D. ($9.95 paper)

MANAGING YOUR PSORIASIS, by Nicholas J. Lowe, M.D. ($10.95 paper, $17.95 cloth)

BUSINESS

TEAMBUILT: Making Teamwork Work, by Mark Sanborn ($19.95 cloth)

DARE TO CHANGE YOUR JOB—AND YOUR LIFE, by Carole Kanchier, Ph.D. ($9.95 paper)

OUT THE ORGANIZATION: New Career Opportunities for the 1990's, by Robert and Madeleine Swain ($12.95 paper)

THE LOYALTY FACTOR: Building Trust in Today's Workplace, by Carol Kinsey Goman, Ph.D. ($9.95 paper)

OFFICE BIOLOGY: Why Tuesday Is the Most Productive Day and Other Relevant Facts for Survival in the Workplace, by Edith Weiner and Arnold Brown ($21.95 cloth)

TWENTYSOMETHING: Managing and Motivating Today's New Work Force, by Lawrence J. Bradford, Ph.D., and Claire Raines, M.A. ($22.95 cloth)

TAKING CONTROL OF YOUR LIFE: The Secrets of Successful Enterprising Women, by Gail Blanke and Kathleen Walas ($17.95 cloth)

SIDE-BY-SIDE STRATEGIES: How Two-Career Couples Can Thrive in the Nineties, by Jane Hershey Cuozzo and S. Diane Graham ($10.95 paper, $19.95 cloth)

WORK WITH ME! How to Make the Most of Office Support Staff, by Betsy Lazary ($9.95 paper)

POSITIVELY OUTRAGEOUS SERVICE: New and Easy Ways to Win Customers for Life, by T. Scott Gross ($14.95 paper)

STEP FORWARD: Sexual Harassment in the Workplace, What You Need to Know, by Susan L. Webb ($9.95 paper)

MIND YOUR OWN BUSINESS: And Keep It in the Family, by Marcy Syms, COO of Syms Corporation ($18.95 cloth)

POSITIVELY OUTRAGEOUS SERVICE AND SHOWMANSHIP, by T. Scott Gross ($12.95 paper)

HOT HEALTH CARE CAREERS, by Margaret T. McNally, R.N., and Phyllis Schneider ($10.95 paper; $17.95 cloth)

SHOCKWAVES, by Susan L. Webb ($9.95 paper, $17.95 cloth)

SELLING YOURSELF, by Kathy Thebo and Joyce Newman ($9.95 paper)

FINANCES and LIFE PLANNING

FINANCIAL SAVVY FOR WOMEN: A Money Book for Women of All Ages, by Dr. Judith Briles ($14.95 paper)

THE DOLLARS AND SENSE OF DIVORCE, by Dr. Judith Briles ($10.95 paper)

AGING PARENTS AND YOU: A Complete Handbook to Help You Help Your Elders Maintain a Healthy, Productive and Independent Life, by Eugenia Anderson-Ellis ($9.95 paper)

CITIES OF OPPORTUNITY: Finding the Best Place to Work, Live and Prosper in the 1990's and Beyond, by Dr. John Tepper Marlin ($13.95 paper, $24.95 cloth)

REAL LIFE 101: The Graduate's Guide to Survival, by Susan Kleinman ($9.95 paper)

BEATING THE AGE GAME, by Jack and Phoebe Ballard ($12.95 paper)

INSPIRATION and MOTIVATION

BREATHING SPACE: Living and Working at a Comfortable Pace in a Sped-Up Society, by Jeff Davidson ($10.95 paper)

CRITICISM IN YOUR LIFE: How to Give It, How to Take It, How to Make It Work for You, by Dr. Deborah Bright ($17.95 cloth)

THE CONFIDENCE FACTOR: How Self-Esteem Can Change Your Life, by Dr. Judith Briles ($9.95 paper, $18.95 cloth)

BEYOND SUCCESS: How Volunteer Service Can Help You Begin Making a Life Instead of Just a Living, by John F. Raynolds III and Eleanor Raynolds, C.B.E. ($19.95 cloth)

HOW TO GET WHAT YOU WANT FROM ALMOST ANYBODY, by T. Scott Gross ($9.95 paper)

DARE TO CONFRONT! How to Intervene When Someone You Care About Has an Alcohol or Drug Problem, by Bob Wright and Deborah George Wright ($17.95 cloth)

FLIGHT PLAN FOR LIVING: The Art of Self-Encouragement, by Patrick O'Dooley ($17.95 cloth)

ON TARGET: Enhance Your Life and Ensure Your Success, by Jeri Sedlar and Rick Miners ($11.95 paper)

MAKING YOUR DREAMS COME TRUE: A Plan for Easily Discovering and Achieving the Life You Want, by Marcia Wieder ($9.95 paper)

CHILD CARE and PARENTING

THE STEPPARENT CHALLENGE: A Primer for Making It Work, by Stephen J. Williams, Sc.D. ($13.95 paper)

BALANCING ACTS! Juggling Love, Work, Family, and Recreation, by Susan Schiffer Stautberg and Marcia L. Worthing ($12.95 paper)

MANAGING YOUR CHILD'S DIABETES, by Robert Wood Johnson IV, Sale Johnson, Casey Johnson, and Susan Kleinman ($10.95 paper)

MANAGING IT ALL: Time-Saving Ideas for Career, Family, Relationships, and Self, by Beverly Benz Treuille and Susan Schiffer Stautberg ($9.95 paper)

NATURE and the ENVIRONMENT

THE SOLUTION TO POLLUTION: 101 Things You Can Do to Clean Up Your Environment, by Laurence Sombke ($7.95 paper)

THE SOLUTION TO POLLUTION IN THE WORKPLACE, by Laurence Sombke, Terry M. Robertson and Elliot M. Kaplan ($9.95 paper)

THE ENVIRONMENTAL GARDENER: The Solution to Pollution for Lawns and Gardens, by Laurence Sombke ($8.95 paper)

OTHER INTERESTS

MANN FOR ALL SEASONS: Wit and Wisdom from The Washington Post's *Judy Mann,* by Judy Mann ($9.95 paper, $19.95 cloth)

GLORIOUS ROOTS: Recipes for Healthy, Tasty Vegetables, by Laurence Sombke ($12.95 paper)

MISS AMERICA: In Pursuit of the Crown, by Ann-Marie Bivans ($19.95 paper, $27.50 cloth; b&w and color photos)

THE BIG APPLE BUSINESS AND PLEASURE GUIDE: 501 Ways to Work Smarter, Play Harder, and Live Better in New York City, by Muriel Siebert and Susan Kleinman ($9.95 paper)

SOMEONE ELSE'S SON, by Alan A. Winter ($18.95 cloth)

FOR YOUNG READERS

WHAT KIDS LIKE TO DO, by Edward Stautberg, Gail Wubbenhorst, Atiya Easterling, and Phyllis Schneider ($7.95 paper)

A TEEN'S GUIDE TO BUSINESS: The Secrets to a Successful Enterprise, by Linda Menzies, Oren S. Jenkins, and Rickell R. Fisher ($7.95 paper)

KIDS WHO MAKE A DIFFERENCE, by Joyce M. Roché and Marie Rodriguez, with Phyllis Schneider ($8.95 paper; with photos)

ROSEY GRIER'S ALL-AMERICAN HEROS: Multicultural Success Stories, by Roosevelt "Rosey" Grier ($9.95 paper; with portrait photos)

ORDER FORM

Print Name_____

Address   _____

             _____

City_____ State_____ Zip_____

Please send me the book(s) indicated below:
_____copy(s) of *THE LIVING HEART GUIDE
        TO EATING OUT* at $9.95 each = $_____

_____copy(s) of *THE LIVING HEART BRAND NAME
        SHOPPER'S GUIDE* at $14.95 each = $_____

        Add $2.00 for postage and handling
            for the first book and $1.50 for
                   each additional book. $_____
                      Total enclosed $_____

Make payment by check or money order payable to Diet
Modification Clinic.
(We cannot accept credit cards.)

Please return to:
   Diet Modification Clinic   Phone: (713) 798-4150
   6565 Fannin, F770   Fax: (713) 798-6409
   Houston, TX 77030

ORDER FORM

Print Name_____

Address   _____

           _____

City_____ State_____ Zip_____

Please send me the book(s) indicated below:
_____copy(s) of *THE LIVING HEART GUIDE
        TO EATING OUT* at $9.95 each = $_____

_____copy(s) of *THE LIVING HEART BRAND NAME
        SHOPPER'S GUIDE* at $14.95 each = $_____

        Add $2.00 for postage and handling
           for the first book and $1.50 for
                 each additional book. $_____
                      Total enclosed $_____

Make payment by check or money order payable to Diet
Modification Clinic.
(We cannot accept credit cards.)

Please return to:
    Diet Modification Clinic   Phone: (713) 798-4150
    6565 Fannin, F770   Fax: (713) 798-6409
    Houston, TX 77030

ORDER FORM

Print Name _____

Address _____

_____

City _____ State _____ Zip _____

Please send me the book(s) indicated below:

_____copy(s) of *THE LIVING HEART GUIDE*
TO EATING OUT at $9.95 each = $_____

_____copy(s) of *THE LIVING HEART BRAND NAME*
SHOPPER'S GUIDE at $14.95 each = $_____

Add $2.00 for postage and handling
for the first book and $1.50 for
each additional book. $_____
Total enclosed $_____

Make payment by check or money order payable to Diet
Modification Clinic.
(We cannot accept credit cards.)

Please return to:
Diet Modification Clinic   Phone: (713) 798-4150
6565 Fannin, F770   Fax: (713) 798-6409
Houston, TX 77030